Obstetrics and Gynecology

Obstetrics and Gynecology:
PreTest® Self-Assessment and Review

Fourth Edition

Edited by

Mark I. Evans, M.D.
Director, Division of Reproductive Genetics
Assistant Professor of Obstetrics and Gynecology
Wayne State University
Hutzel Hospital
Detroit, Michigan

McGraw-Hill Book Company
Health Professions Division
PreTest Series

New York   St. Louis   San Francisco
Auckland   Bogotá   Hamburg
Lisbon   London   Madrid   Mexico
Milan   Montreal   New Delhi   Panama
Paris   San Juan   São Paulo   Singapore
Sydney   Tokyo   Toronto

Notice

Medicine is an ever-changing science. As new research and clinical experience broaden our knowledge, changes in treatment and drug therapy are required. The editor and the publisher of this work have made every effort to ensure that the drug dosage schedules herein are accurate and in accord with the standards accepted at the time of publication. Readers are advised, however, to check the product information sheet included in the package of each drug they plan to administer to be certain that changes have not been made in the recommended dose or in the contraindications for administration. This recommendation is of particular importance in connection with new or infrequently used drugs.

Library of Congress Cataloging in Publication Data
Main entry under title:

Obstetrics and gynecology: PreTest self-assessment and review.

Bibliography: p.
  1. Gynecology—Examinations, questions, etc.
2. Obstetrics—Examinations, questions, etc.   I. Evans,
Mark I. [DNLM: 1. Gynecology—examination questions.
2. Obstetrics—examination questions.   WP 18 014]
RG111.037   1987   618'.076   86-33783
ISBN 0-07-051013-X

This book was set in Times Roman by Waldman Graphics, Inc.; the editors were Eileen J. Scott and Bruce MacGregor; the production supervisor was Clara B. Stanley.
Semline, Inc., was printer and binder.

2 3 4 5 6 7 8 9 0   SEMSEM   8 9 4 3 2 1 0 9 8

ISBN 0-07-051013-X

Contents

Introduction

Obstetrics and Gynecology: PreTest Self-Assessment and Review, 4th Ed.,
has been designed to provide medical students, as well as physicians, with
a comprehensive and convenient instrument for self-assessment and review
within the field of obstetrics and gynecology. The 500 questions provided
have been designed to parallel the format and degree of difficulty of the
questions contained in Part II of the National Board of Medical Examiners
examinations, the Federation Licensing Examination (FLEX), and the Foreign Medical Graduate Examination in the Medical Sciences (FMGEMS).

Each question in the book is accompanied by an answer, a paragraph
explanation, and a specific page reference to either a current journal article,
a textbook, or both. A bibliography that lists all the sources used in the book
follows the last chapter.

Perhaps the most effective way to use this book is to allow yourself one
minute to answer each question in a given chapter; as you proceed, indicate
your answer beside each question. By following this suggestion, you will
be approximating the time limits imposed by the board examinations previously mentioned.

When you have finished answering the questions in a chapter, you should
then spend as much time as you need verifying your answers and carefully
reading the explanations. Although you should pay special attention to the
explanations for the questions you answered incorrectly, you should read
every explanation. The explanations have been designed to reinforce and
supplement the information tested by the questions. If, after reading the
explanations for a given chapter, you feel you need still more information
about the material covered, you should consult and study the references
indicated.

BIOLOGY
AND PHYSIOLOGY
OF REPRODUCTION

Anatomy, Genetics, Embryology, and Congenital Anomalies

DIRECTIONS: Each question below contains five suggested responses. Select the **one best** response to each question.

1. In a screening program for neural tube defects using maternal serum alpha-fetoprotein (MSAFP), the next step following two successive elevated MSAFP blood tests should be

(A) a third MSAFP test
(B) ultrasound examination
(C) amniocentesis
(D) amniography
(E) recommendation of termination

2. The most important indication for surgical repair of a double uterus is

(A) habitual abortion
(B) dysmenorrhea
(C) menometrorrhagia
(D) dyspareunia
(E) premature delivery

3. The most common cause of ambiguous genitalia in infants is

(A) chromosomal nondisjunction
(B) gonadal dysgenesis
(C) adrenal hyperplasia
(D) mosaicism
(E) testicular feminization

4. The third trimester fetus of a mother with a balanced 13/13 translocation would have what likelihood of having an abnormal chromosome karyotype?

(A) 2 percent
(B) 10 percent
(C) 25 percent
(D) 50 percent
(E) 100 percent

5. Achondroplasia is characterized by which of the following statements?

(A) The inheritance pattern is autosomal recessive
(B) Mutation accounts for 90 percent of all cases
(C) Cesarean section is rarely necessary
(D) Affected women rarely live to the reproductive age
(E) None of the above

6. A 42-year-old woman undergoes a Marshall-Marchetti-Krantz operation for true urinary stress incontinence. The jack-knife position in which the knees are bent and abducted laterally is used during the procedure. Postoperatively, the patient complains of foot-drop and loss of sensation on the dorsal apsect of her right foot. The nerve most likely to have been injured during this operation is the

(A) obturator
(B) internal pudendal
(C) common peroneal
(D) ilioinguinal
(E) genitofemoral

7. The most common defect of the adrenogenital syndrome is

(A) idiopathic
(B) 11-hydroxylase deficiency
(C) 17-hydroxylase deficiency
(D) 21-hydroxylase deficiency
(E) 3-beta-o1-dehydrogenase
    deficiency

8. The ultrasound image below is representative of

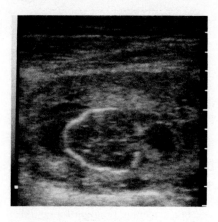

(A) a cystic hygroma
(B) an encephalocele
(C) hydrocephalus
(D) anencephaly
(E) none of the above

DIRECTIONS: Each question below contains four suggested responses of which **one or more** is correct. Select

A	if	**1, 2, and 3**	are correct
B	if	**1 and 3**	are correct
C	if	**2 and 4**	are correct
D	if	**4**	is correct
E	if	**1, 2, 3, and 4**	are correct

9. The karyotypes associated with Turner's syndrome include

(1) 46,XXr
(2) 46,XXp-
(3) 46,Xi(Xq)
(4) 46,X,i(Xp)

10. In patients with carcinoma of the vulva, lymphatic drainage characteristically

(1) is to the periaortic nodes
(2) is to the superficial inguinal lymph nodes
(3) bypasses the deep femoral lymph nodes
(4) is from the clitoral region to the deep femoral lymph nodes

11. The advantages of transverse abdominal incisions include

(1) a decreased incidence of incisional hernias
(2) the requirement of only light general anesthesia
(3) a scar that can be cosmetically hidden
(4) easy access to the upper abdomen for bowel surgery

12. A carrier of a balanced 14/21 (D/G) translocation is described by which of the following statements?

(1) Amniocentesis or chorionic villus sampling can detect offspring who have translocation Down syndrome as well as those who are balanced carriers
(2) Karyotype analysis would reveal 45 chromosomes in each cell
(3) Chromosome studies of members of a carrier's family are indicated to detect others at risk for having children with Down syndrome
(4) The risk for bearing children who have Down syndrome is the same whether the husband or the wife is the carrier

13. A group of congenital anomalies known collectively as Potter syndrome includes renal agenesis (or other renal anomalies) and pulmonary hypoplasia. Other anomalies associated with Potter syndrome include

(1) hydrocephaly
(2) amnion nodosum
(3) cleft palate
(4) oligohydramnios

SUMMARY OF DIRECTIONS

A	B	C	D	E
1,2,3 only	1,3 only	2,4 only	4 only	All are correct

14. Diseases that have a positive correlation between maternal infection during pregnancy and congenital anomalies in the fetus include

(1) rubella
(2) mumps
(3) cytomegalovirus
(4) influenza

15. Individuals with the karyotype 45,X are likely to have

(1) a webbed neck, shield chest, high-arched palate, and low-set ears
(2) lymphedema of the extremities at birth
(3) a high incidence of diabetes mellitus
(4) mothers who are over 35 years of age

16. True statements regarding ambiguous genitalia include which of the following?

(1) A karyotype must be obtained
(2) It is a medical emergency at birth
(3) It is sometimes associated with a history of a previous sibling with congenital adrenal hyperplasia (CAH)
(4) A thorough physical examination can usually decide the true sex

17. Advantages of chorionic villus sampling (CVS) over amniocentesis include that

(1) CVS can be performed earlier in pregnancy
(2) the results of CVS are usually available faster
(3) genetic terminations in the first trimester after CVS are safer than terminations in the second trimester after other tests
(4) CVS has a lower complication rate than amniocentesis

18. Which of the following conditions can be diagnosed by DNA analysis of amniotic fluid cells on chorionic villi?

(1) Sickle cell anemia
(2) Duchenne muscular dystrophy
(3) Hemophilia A
(4) Tay-Sachs disease

19. True statements about a pregnant woman who has phenylketonuria include which of the following?

(1) If the father carries the gene, the risk that the child will be affected is 25 percent
(2) If the father carries the gene, amniocentesis or chorionic villus sampling and selective abortion can avert the birth of affected children
(3) Individuals with phenylketonuria rarely survive to the reproductive years
(4) Genetically normal children born to mothers who have phenylketonuria are frequently mentally retarded

20. A bicornuate uterus (bicornis unicollis) is associated with

(1) failure of complete fusion of the
müllerian duct system
(2) an increase in obstetrical complications
(3) an increase in urinary tract anomalies
(4) cervical and vaginal malformations

DIRECTIONS: Each group of questions below consists of lettered headings followed by a set of numbered items. For each numbered item select the **one** lettered heading with which it is **most** closely associated. Each lettered heading may be used **once, more than once, or not at all.**

Questions 21–23

For each situation below, select the appropriate inheritance pattern.

(A) Autosomal dominant
(B) Autosomal recessive
(C) X-linked recessive
(D Codominant
(E) Multifactorial

21. Glucose-6-phosphate dehydrogenase deficiency

22. Neurofibromatosis

23. Haplotypes

Questions 24–28

For each structure below, select its embryological origin.

(A) Genital tubercle
(B) Genital swellings
(C) Urogenital sinus
(D) Urethral folds
(E) Müllerian ducts

24. Labia minora

25. Labia majora

26. Clitoris

27. Lower one third of vagina

28. Fallopian tubes

Questions 29–33

Match the following female structures with their male homologues.

(A) Gubernaculum testis
(B) Prostate gland
(C) Scrotum
(D) Vas deferens
(E) Phallus

29. Paraurethral glands

30. Labia majora

31. Round ligament

32. Gartner's duct

33. Clitoris

Questions 34–38

For each description that follows, select the blood vessel with which it is most likely to be associated.

(A) Uterine vein
(B) Right ovarian vein
(C) Left ovarian vein
(D) Uterine artery
(E) Ovarian artery

34. Arises from the anterior branch of the hypogastric artery

35. Drains into the internal iliac veins

36. Drains into the inferior vena cava

37. Arises from the abdominal aorta

38. Drains into the left renal vein

Questions 39–45

For each condition that follows, select the study that would be helpful in detecting that condition in utero.

(A) Fetal chromosome count
(B) Fetal sex determination
(C) Amniotic fluid level of alpha-fetoprotein
(D) Enzyme analysis of cultured amniotic fluid cells
(E) None of the above

39. Meningomyelocele

40. Neurofibromatosis

41. Tay-Sachs disease

42. Klinefelter syndrome

43. Hurler syndrome

44. Translocation Down syndrome

45. Hydrocephaly (without associated spinal cord defects)

Anatomy, Genetics, Embryology, and Congenital Anomalies

Answers

1. The answer is B. *(Gastel, p 43.)* The recommended sequence for a MSAFP screening program for 1000 hypothetical patients would have 50 with an elevated (2.5 multiples of the normal median) first MSAFP test. About 30 would demonstrate elevated levels in the second MSAFP test. Next, a thorough ultrasound examination should reveal about 15 patients with an obvious reason for the elevation: e.g., anencephaly, twins, wrong gestational age of fetus, or fetal demise. About 15 patients with no obvious cause should be offered amniocentesis. Of these 15 about 1 to 2 will have elevated amniotic fluid AFP confirmed by acetylcholinesterase. Such patients will have a greater than 99 percent chance of having a neural tube defect or other serious malformation. Amniography is an outmoded procedure in which radiopaque dye is injected into the amniotic cavity for the purpose of taking x-rays. Under no circumstances whatsoever should termination be recommended on the basis of MSAFP tests alone.

2. The answer is A. *(Mattingly, ed 6. pp 367–369.)* Habitual abortion is the most important indication for surgical treatment of women who have a double uterus. The abortion rate in women who have a double uterus is two to three times greater than that of the general population. Therefore, women who present with habitual abortion should be evaluated by hysterosalpingography to detect a possible double uterus. Dysmenorrhea, premature delivery, dyspareunia, and menometrorrhagia are other, less important indications for surgical intervention.

3. The answer is C. *(Evans, pp 130–137.)* Although congenital adrenal hyperplasia (CAH) affects both sexes, it more often is recognized in female neonates. CAH accounts for approximately 50 percent of all cases of ambiguous sexual differentiation. Despite its genetic origin, congenital adrenal hyperplasia is not associated with karyotypic abnormalities. The most typical abnormality of external genitalia is clitoral enlargement, which is usually accompanied by some degree of hypospadias and labioscrotal fusion.

4.   The answer is E. *(Thompson, ed 4. pp 121–126.)* Carriers of balanced translocations of the same chromosome are phenotypically normal. However, in the process of gamete formation (either sperm or ova), the translocated chromosome cannot divide and therefore the meiosis products end up with either two copies or no copies of the particular chromosome. In the former case, fertilization leads to trisomy of that chromosome. Many trisomies are lethal in utero. Trisomies of 13, 18, and 21 lead to classic syndromes. In the latter case, a monosomy is produced, and all except for monosomy X (Turner syndrome) are lethal in utero.

5.   The answer is B. *(Smith, ed 3. pp 248–251.)* Achondroplasia, a congenital disorder of cartilage formation characterized by dwarfism, is associated with an autosomal dominant pattern of inheritance. However, mutation accounts for 90 percent of all cases of the disorder. Affected women almost always require cesarean section because of the distorted shape of their pelves. Women who have achondroplasia and receive adequate treatment for its associated complications, including the neurological signs of cord compression due to spinal deformity, generally have a normal life expectancy.

6.   The answer is C. *(Mattingly, ed 6. pp 43–49.)* The jack-knife position described in the question commonly gives rise to injury of the sciatic or peroneal nerve through the overstretching of the nerve over the sacrospinous ligament. The symptoms of footdrop and loss of sensation over the dorsal aspect of the foot classically accompany peroneal nerve injury. The ilioinguinal and genitofemoral nerves traverse the inguinal canal together with the round ligament. The obturator nerve, which runs along the lateral wall of the pelvis, can be damaged by deep retractors and during radical pelvic surgery. It supplies all the adducter muscles of the thigh as well as provides the sensory supply to the medial aspects of the thigh. The internal pudendal nerve is derived from S_2-S_3 and supplies the vulva and perineum.

7.   The answer is D. *(Speroff, ed 3. pp 344–345.)* This enzyme block is the most frequent cause of sexual ambiguity and the most frequent endocrine cause of neonatal death. Serum 17-hydroxyprogesterone and urinary pregnanetriol are elevated. Neonatal complications are related to salt loss because of inadequate mineralocorticoid production in some of these infants.

8.   The answer is B. *(Jeanty, pp 105–106.)* An encephalocele is an outpouching of neural tissue through a defect in the skull. A cystic hygroma, with which it can often be confused on ultrasound, emerges from the base of the neck with an intact skull present. Hydrocephalus is related to the size of the lateral ventricles and anencephaly would require absence of a much larger proportion of the skull with diminished neural tissues.

9.   The answer is A (1, 2, 3). *(Therman, pp 130–132.)* Although monosomy of the X chromosome (45,X) is the most common karyotype of patients who have Turner syndrome, a variety of structural abnormalities of the X chromosome in addition to mosaics may be found in patients who have this disorder. Comparison of chromosomal abnormalities and phenotypic features in individuals who have gonadal dysgenesis indicates that the short stature and other clinical findings of Turner phenotype are associated with loss of the short arm of one X chromosome. Of the karyotypes listed in the question, all involve monosomy for a portion of the short arm of the X chromosome except 46,X,i(Xp). Individuals who have this karyotype have only one normal X chromosome; their other X chromosome, composed of a duplication of the normal short arm, is called an isochromosome. In essence, they are monosomic for the long arm of the X and trisomic for the short arm. This karyotype is associated with gonadal dysgenesis but not with the phenotypic features characteristic of individuals who have Turner's syndrome.

10.   The answer is C (2, 4). *(Mattingly, ed 6. pp 717–718.)* An important feature of the lymphatic drainage of the vulva is the existence of drainage across the midline. The vulva drains first into the superficial inguinal lymph nodes, then into the deep femoral nodes, and finally into the external iliac lymph nodes. The clinical significance of this sequence for patients with carcinoma of the vulva is that the iliac nodes are probably free of the disease if the deep femoral nodes are not involved. Unlike the lymphatic drainage from the rest of the vulva, the drainage from the clitoral region bypasses the superficial inguinal nodes and passes directly to the deep femoral nodes. Thus, while the superficial nodes will usually also have metastases when the deep femoral nodes are implicated, it is possible for only the deep nodes to be involved if the carcinoma is in the midline near the clitoris.

11.   The answer is B (1, 3). *(Mattingly, ed 6. pp 157–159.)* Benefits of a low transverse abdominal incision are a decreased incidence of incisional hernias and cosmetic placement of the scar near the edge of the pubic hairline. The use of light anesthesia is contraindicated because it provides poor muscle relaxation. Bowel surgery is best approached with a vertical incision, especially if a colostomy is anticipated.

12.   The answer is A (1, 2, 3). *(Thompson, ed 4. pp 118–119, 122.)* Individuals who are carriers of a balanced D/G translocation have 45 chromosomes in each cell; one D-group and one G-group chromosome have fused, forming a chromosome that resembles a member of the C group. The risk for giving birth to children who have translocation Down's syndrome is substantially higher if the wife is the carrier (10 to 12 percent) than if the husband is the carrier (2 to 3 percent). Amniocentesis can determine whether the offspring will be unaffected, will carry the translocation, or will have the disease. Because a D/G translocation can be inherited from a parent (approximately 50 percent are familial), chromosome studies of family members are recommended.

13. The answer is C (2, 4). *(Pritchard, ed 17. pp 465, 804.)* An infant with Potter's syndrome generally has a breech presentation. After birth, the baby is never able to ventilate adequately. These infants rarely survive more than a few hours. The primary lesion in Potter syndrome is thought to be renal. Because of renal agenesis, urine output is impossible, and oligohydramnios results. Oligohydramnios is believed to lead to pulmonary hypoplasia, because lack of amniotic fluid somehow restricts normal lung development. The characteristic facial anomalies (large, low-set ears and flattened nose) are thought to be related to pressure on the face increased by a lack of cushioning amniotic fluid. The diagnosis of Potter syndrome has been made antenatally with the aid of ultrasonography. Demonstration of a fetal bladder that fills and empties should rule out Potter syndrome. The absence of evidence of a bladder, despite repeated ultrasonographic examinations, would be compatible with the diagnosis. Amnion nodosum, another common finding in Potter syndrome, consists of multiple opaque nodules in the amnion. Their etiology is not clear, but they represent fetal squames that have become "parasitic" on the membranes.

14. The answer is B (1,3). *(Burrow, ed 2. pp 333–350.)* Rubella syndrome in the newborn secondary to rubella infection during pregnancy (especially, not exclusively, during the first trimester) is well known. Although cytomegalovirus infection is less familiar, it is thought to cause congenital anomalies in about 500 newborns every year in the United States. The abnormalities are usually in the central nervous system and include microcephaly, cerebral calcifications, deafness, and other mental and motor disabilities. Although there have been some suggestions that influenza epidemics have led to a subsequent rise in the incidence of childhood leukemia, this relationship has not been established; in fact, there is no proof that influenza is associated with any anomalies. Mumps is relatively common during pregnancy, but prospective studies have failed to show any associated congenital anomalies.

15. The answer is A (1, 2, 3). *(Smith, ed 3. pp 72–75.)* Individuals with a 45,X karyotype have Turner syndrome (gonadal dysgenesis), a disorder in phenotypic females characterized by a variety of physical abnormalities. In addition to those listed in the question, pigmented nevi, a short fourth metacarpal, wide-set nipples, and renal and cardiovascular anomalies are common. Lymphedema presents as puffiness of the hands and feet at birth. Diabetes mellitus is also prevalent among these children. Gonadal dysgenesis, unlike other chromosomal abnormalities, is not related to maternal age.

16. The answer is A (1, 2, 3). *(Kase, p 237).* Ambiguous genitalia at birth are a medical emergency not only for psychologic reassurance for the parents but also because hirsute female infants with congenital adrenal hyperplasia (CAH) may die if undiagnosed. CAH is an autosomally inherited disease of adrenal failure that causes hyponatremia and hyperkalemia because of lack of mineralocorticoids. Although a thorough physical examination is helpful, especially for inguinal testes, other tests that are required include a karyotype, serum electrolytes, and blood or urine assays for progesterone, 17 α-hydroxy-progesterone, and androgens such as dehydroepiandrosterone sulfate. Radiology studies are usually not needed but a laparotomy is sometimes necessary for ectopic gonadectomy.

17. The answer is A (1,2,3) *(Evans, ed 3. pp 137–139.)* Chorionic villus sampling (CVS) has many theoretical and practical advantages over amniocentesis, including its earlier performance and quicker results. Suction VIPs during the first trimester are safer than prostaglandin and other second-trimester techniques. However, CVS does have a somewhat higher complication rate. In the most experienced hands, genetic amniocentesis probably carries about a 1/400 risk and CVS probably has a 1/100 to 1/200 risk.

18. The answer is A (1,2,3). *(Evans, ed 3. pp 140–142.)* Through the use of restriction fragment length polymorphisms (RFLPs), it is often possible to determine from which parent segments of DNA are inherited. In an ''informative'' family— one in which the parents are heterozygous at the locus in question—it is possible to predict to a high degree of certainty whether or not the fetus will be affected with many disorders, including sickle cell anemia, hemophilias A and B, and Duchenne's muscular dystrophy. The diagnosis of Tay-Sachs disease is made by enzyme assay of hexosaminidase A. The number of conditions that can be diagnosed by RFLPs is growing very rapidly.

19. The answer is C (2,4). *(Smith, ed 3. p 434.)* If a woman who has phenylketonuria (PKU), which is an autosomal recessive disorder, marries a carrier for this disease, the chance that offspring will be affected is 50 percent. Phenylketonuria can now be detected prenatally through the use of molecular techniques. Screening of newborns and early institution of low-phenylalanine diets have made it possible for affected individuals to reach adulthood. It has become apparent that a high frequency of mental retardation exists in children of mothers who have phenylketonuria, even if these children do not themselves have the disease. Retardation in these children presumably is related to intrauterine exposure to high phenylalanine levels in the maternal blood. Whether or not a mother with PKU can be ''compelled'' to follow a diet for the sake of the developing fetus will be a significant ethical debate of the late 1980s.

20. The answer is A (1, 2, 3). *(Mattingly, ed 6. pp 365–378.)* Failure of fusion of the müllerian ducts can give rise to the several types of uterine anomalies of which uterus bicornis unicollis is a representative type. This condition is associated with higher obstetrical complications, such as an increase in the rate of second-trimester abortion and premature labor. If the pregnancies go to term, malpresentations such as breech and transverse lies are frequent. Also, prolonged labor, which is probably due to inadequate muscle development in the uterus, increased bleeding, and a higher incidence of fetal anomalies caused by defective implantation of the placenta all occur far more commonly than in normal pregnancies. An intravenous pyelogram is mandatory in the workup of patients with uterine anomalies as there is an associated higher incidence of urinary tract anomalies. In uterus bicornis unicollis, there is a single cervix with a normal vagina.

21–23. The answers are: 21-C, 22-A, 23-D. *(Smith, ed 3. pp 377–379. Thompson, ed 4. pp 44–65, 216–224.)* Glucose-6-phosphate dehydrogenase (G6PD) deficiency is X-linked recessive and is found predominantly in males of African and Mediterranean origin. Although the causes of clinical manifestations in G6PD deficiency are multifactorial (e.g., sulfa drugs), the inheritance is not.

Neurofibromatosis, whose occurrence is often sporadic (i.e., a spontaneous mutation in 50 percent), is inherited as an autosomal dominant once the gene is in a family. The severity of the condition can be quite variable even within the same family.

The HLA antigens (four from each parent) are all expressed and therefore do not show any "dominance" in their expression. Certain combinations of haplotypes are associated with some disease conditions (such as 21-hydroxylase deficiency congenital adrenal hyperplasia) in that they occur much more commonly than would be expected by chance; however, such associations do not, alone, define inheritance.

24–28. The answers are: 24-D, 25-B, 26-A, 27-C, 28-E. *(Mattingly, ed 6. pp 345–349.)* In the female, the urethral folds give rise to the labia minora, while the labia majora are formed from the genital swellings. It is believed that the development of external genitalia is dependent on the presence of hormones during the intrauterine period. With the absence of androgens and the inducer substance in females, the wolffian duct system regresses while the external genitalia develop under the influence of estrogen from both maternal and placental sources.

In the male, the genital tubercle gives rise to the phallus, while in the female it elongates minimally to form the clitoris. Clitoral hypertrophy can occur in conditions in which there is an abnormally high level of circulating androgens during the critical phase of development of the external genitalia. Congenital adrenal hyperplasia and mixed gonadal dysgenesis are two clinical situations that may present with clitoral hypertrophy.

There are several theories to explain the embryological origin of the vagina; however, it is generally accepted that the upper two thirds of the vagina are of müllerian duct origin while the lower one third is of urogenital sinus origin, which seems to explain in part the congenital anomalies that arise in this anatomical region. A common anomaly of urogenital sinus origin is imperforate hymen, which is easily treated by hymenotomy. Congenital absence of the vagina is an anomaly of müllerian duct origin and, as such, usually involves an absence of only the upper two thirds of the vagina, as well as an absence of the uterus and fallopian tubes in most cases.

In the female, the müllerian ducts give rise to the fallopian tubes, uterus, and cervix. Imperfect fusion of the müllerian ducts can give rise to a whole spectrum of uterine anomalies, which may be associated with clinical entities like habitual abortions, prematurity, and fetal malpositions. Patients with proven müllerian duct anomalies should have an intravenous pyelogram to rule out urinary tract anomalies that may be present.

29–33. The answers are: 29-B, 30-C, 31-A, 32-D, 33-E. *(Pritchard, ed 17. p 28.)* The male homologue of the round ligament is the gubernaculum testis. It is a cordlike structure extending from the lower pole of the testis to the scrotum. Abnormalities of this structure are associated with maldescent of the testes. The round ligaments play a minor role in support of the uterus.

The prostate gland corresponds with the paraurethral glands in females. Clinically, these glands and their canals, which open into both the urethra and the Skene's ducts, can serve as a reservoir for gonococcal infections. Also these glands can become cystic with chronic infections, giving rise to suburethral diverticula.

In the embryological development of the external genitalia of the female, the urethral folds and the genital swellings do not fuse, giving rise to the labia minora and the labia majora, respectively. The contrary is true in the male, as the urethral folds fuse to form the penis, while the scrotum is formed by the fusion of the genital swellings.

The vas deferens and Gartner's duct are both derived from the wolffian duct system. Cysts of Gartner's duct, when present, are usually found along the antero-lateral wall of the vagina. They are usually asymptomatic and rarely require surgical intervention.

Embryologically, the male phallus and the female clitoris both arise from the genital tubercle. Hypertrophy of the clitoris can occur if there is a high level of androgens present during the early development of the external genitalia.

34–38. The answers are: 34-D, 35-A, 36-B, 37-E, 38-C. *(Mattingly, ed 6. pp 49–52.)* The blood supply of the pelvic organs and musculature is derived primarily from the hypogastric artery. The uterine artery arises from the anterior division of the hypogastric artery and supplies the vagina, uterus, and fallopian tubes. The bladder is also supplied by the vesical branches of the hypogastric artery, which terminates as the internal pudendal artery supplying the perineum, labia, and clitoris, as well as the thigh muscles. The uterine veins, which drain into the internal iliac veins, generally follow the course of the uterine arteries. Together, they course superiorly to the ureters along the base of the broad ligaments.

The two ovarian veins follow different courses. The right ovarian vein drains into the inferior vena cava just below the level of the right renal vein, while the left ovarian vein drains into the left renal vein. The right ovarian vein may become distended during pregnancy, causing partial obstruction of the ureter proximal to its course. This has been postulated to be a cause of right hydronephrosis in pregnancy. The ovarian artery arises from the abdominal aorta. It courses through the infundibulopelvic ligament and supplies the ovary and the fallopian tube.

A thorough understanding of the above-mentioned relationships is essential in gynecological surgery, especially in cases of hemorrhage requiring hypogastric artery ligation.

39–45. The answers are: 39-C, 40-E, 41-D, 42-A, 43-D, 44-E, 45-E. *(Evans, ed 3. pp 130–144.)* Aneuploidy can be detected simply by counting fetal chromosomes; however, nonbanded karyotypes are no longer adequate in modern genetics. The diagnosis of aneuploid disorders, such as Klinefelter syndrome (47,XXY) and trisomy 21 (classic Down syndrome) can be confirmed by karyotype. Because individuals who have translocation Down syndrome have 46 chromosomes, a chromosome count per se would be misleading; modern chromosome-banding techniques, however, can demonstrate this abnormality during analysis of the karyotype. Although neurofibromatosis is an inherited, autosomal dominant disorder, it cannot be detected prenatally at this time.

Meningomyelocele and other open neural-tube defects have markedly elevated amniotic fluid levels of alpha-fetoprotein, probably as a result of the transudation of this protein across the membrane covering the defect. If a neural-tube defect is completely covered with skin, however, the alpha-fetoprotein level may be within normal limits; an example of such closed defects is hydrocephaly that is not associated with spinal cord lesions.

Tay-Sachs disease results from a defect in the synthesis of hexosaminidase A. Hurler syndrome is caused by a deficiency of the enzyme α-iduronidase. Both disorders can be detected by enzyme analysis of cultured fetal cells grown from amniotic fluid or chorionic villi.

Puberty, Menstruation, Menopause, Sexuality, and Conception

DIRECTIONS: Each question below contains five suggested responses. Select the **one best** response to each question.

46. Follicle-stimulating hormone is elaborated by

(A) chromophobe cells of the adenohypophysis
(B) basophilic cells of the adenohypophysis
(C) acidophilic cells of the adenohypophysis
(D) theca interna cells
(E) none of the above

47. In what percentage of girls with precocious puberty is this constitutional (nonorganic) in origin?

(A) 10 percent
(B) 25 percent
(C) 30 percent
(D) 50 percent
(E) 90 percent

48. Peripheral conversion of estrogen precursors in the obese patient after menopause results primarily in the formation of

(A) estriol
(B) estradiol
(C) estrone
(D) androstenedione
(E) dehydroepiandrosterone

49. The ovaries of an infant at birth contain oocytes that have progressed to

(A) prophase of the first meiotic division
(B) formation of oogonia
(C) maturation
(D) anaphase of the second meiotic division
(E) none of the above

50. In the testis, which of the following can be **directly** influenced by luteinizing hormone (LH)?

(A) Leydig cells
(B) Sertoli cells
(C) Leydig cells and Sertoli cells
(D) Leydig cells and seminiferous tubules
(E) Sertoli cells and seminiferous tubules

51. Which of the following allows for the **earliest** determination of probable pregnancy?

(A) Pelvic examination
(B) Ultrasonography
(C) Basal temperature curves
(D) Hemagglutination-inhibition test
(E) Assay of the serum beta subunit of human chorionic gonadotropin

52. If a man received a severe thermal trauma to his testes, his previously normal sperm count would become depressed in about

(A) 1 day
(B) 7 days
(C) 30 days
(D) 75 days
(E) 100 days

53. The average blood loss resulting from menstruation is

(A) 10 to 15 ml
(B) 25 to 50 ml
(C) 75 to 100 ml
(D) 101 to 125 ml
(E) 130 to 150 ml

54. According to Masters and Johnson, factors that increase the likelihood of female orgasm during intercourse include

(A) a larger clitoral glans
(B) a clitoris located closer to the vaginal introitus
(C) erection of the clitoral shaft
(D) male superior coital position
(E) none of the above

55. Which of the following contraceptive methods are correctly ranked in terms of decreasing effectiveness?

(A) Oral contraceptives, diaphragm, IUD, spermicides, rhythm
(B) IUD, oral contraceptives, diaphragm, spermicides, rhythm
(C) Rhythm, oral contraceptives, IUD, diaphragm, spermicides
(D) Oral contraceptives, IUD, spermicides, diaphragm, rhythm
(E) Oral contraceptives, IUD, diaphragm, spermicides, rhythm

56. All the following are major regulators of the menstrual cycle EXCEPT

(A) estradiol
(B) luteinizing hormone (LH)
(C) progesterone
(D) human chorionic gonadotropin (HCG)
(E) follicle-stimulating hormone (FSH)

DIRECTIONS: Each question below contains four suggested responses of which **one or more** is correct. Select

A	if	**1, 2, and 3**	are correct
B	if	**1 and 3**	are correct
C	if	**2 and 4**	are correct
D	if	**4**	is correct
E	if	**1, 2, 3, and 4**	are correct

57. True statements regarding vaginismus include that it is

(1) a reflex spastic involuntary contraction of the vaginal outlet
(2) detectable on pelvic examination
(3) associated with secondary impotence in the male partner
(4) in part treated with vaginal dilators

58. Physiological processes that are estrogen-dependent in women include which of the following?

(1) Menses
(2) Vaginal cornification
(3) Appearance of axillary hair
(4) Cervical mucus formation

59. Causes of delayed puberty include

(1) anorexia nervosa
(2) syndromes of androgen excess
(3) gonadal dysgenesis
(4) chronic disease

60. Sequelae of vasectomy include

(1) varicocele
(2) sperm granuloma
(3) torsion of the testis
(4) sperm antibodies

61. Postmenopausal patients may need special attention to which of the following problems?

(1) Vaginitis
(2) Depression
(3) Osteoporosis
(4) Sexual dysfunction

62. Significant components of vaginal lubrication include

(1) fluid from Skene's glands
(2) mucus produced by endocervical glands
(3) viscous fluid from Bartholin's glands
(4) transudate-like material from the vaginal walls

63. Characteristics of the gonadotropins (FSH and LH) include

(1) stimulation of the production of primordial follicles
(2) stimulation of the production of estrogen by thecal cells
(3) stimulation of the production of spermatozoa and testosterone in men who have hypopituitarism
(4) a glycoprotein structure

SUMMARY OF DIRECTIONS

A	B	C	D	E
1,2,3 only	1,3 only	2,4 only	4 only	All are correct

64. Menopause is characterized by which of the following?

(1) Occurrence generally at age 40 to 45
(2) Absence of menses for 6 to 12 months in a woman over 45 years old
(3) Invariable appearance of hot flushes prior to menopause
(4) Elevated FSH and LH levels

65. Physiological actions occurring during the plateau phase of sexual excitement in women include

(1) areolar tumescence
(2) systolic blood pressure elevations
(3) involuntary skeletal muscle contractions
(4) involuntary contractions of the rectal sphincter

66. Essential precursors of the Δ^5-3β-hydroxy pathway include

(1) pregnenolone
(2) dehydroepiandrosterone
(3) estradiol
(4) progesterone

67. The contraceptive effect of birth control pills containing both synthetic estrogen and progestin is related to the

(1) inhibition of ovulation
(2) impaired penetrability of sperm into the cervical mucus
(3) atrophic changes of the endometrium impairing implantation
(4) uterotubal hypermotility impairing sperm transport

68. Cholesterol can be synthesized from acetate by which of the following organs?

(1) Ovary
(2) Adrenal gland
(3) Testis
(4) Placenta

69. Polypeptide structure and direct inducement of hormonal changes in target organs are characteristics of which of the following hormones?

(1) Prolactin
(2) Growth hormone
(3) Chorionic somatomammotropin
(4) Thyrotropin

DIRECTIONS: Each group of questions below consists of lettered headings followed by a set of numbered items. For each numbered item select the **one** lettered heading with which it is **most** closely associated. Each lettered heading may be used **once, more than once, or not at all.**

Questions 70–74

Match each action listed below with the appropriate enzyme.

(A) Adenylcyclase
(B) 5 α-Reductase
(C) 17β-Hydroxylase
(D) 20-Hydroxylase
(E) 21-Dehydroxylase

70. Is activated by LH

71. Converts androstenedione to testosterone

72. Converts testosterone to dihydro-testosterone

73. Catalyzes the first step in the production of hormonal steroids from cholesterol

74. Causes massive adrenal enlargement when congenitally deficient, is associated with poor survival of the affected infants, and can lead to the formation of female genitalia in genotypically male infants

Puberty, Menstruation, Menopause, Sexuality, and Conception

Answers

46. The answer is B. *(Jones, ed 10. p 47.)* Luteinizing hormone (LH) and follicle-stimulating hormone (FSH) are synthesized, stored, and secreted from the basophilic cells of the anterior pituitary. It appears that a single cell type makes both LH and FSH.

47. The answer is E. *(Speroff, ed 3. pp 370–374.)* In constitutional sexual precocity there is premature maturation of the hypothalamic-pituitary-ovarian axis, resulting in production of gonadotropins and sex steroids. This is usually a diagnosis of exclusion and deserves long-term follow-up for detection of possible organic problems.

48. The answer is C. *(Speroff, ed 3. p 103.)* The circulating level of estrone in the postmenopausal woman is higher than that of estradiol. Estrone is principally derived from peripheral conversion of androstenedione in adipose tissue. The percent conversion of androstenedione to estrogen correlates with body weight.

49. The answer is A. *(Speroff, ed 3. p 103.)* Evidence of nuclear maturation is first seen at about 15 weeks of gestation. The oogonia are transformed to oocytes as they enter the first meiotic division and arrest in prophase. The second meiotic division is not completed until fertilization.

50. The answer is A. *(Wilson, ed 7. pp 171–172.)* In the testis, Leydig cells produce testosterone, Sertoli cells primarily provide structural support and nutrition, and seminiferous tubules produce sperm. Leydig cells are under the influence of luteinizing hormone (LH) in a negative-feedback relationship. Testosterone produced by Leydig cells regulates spermatogenesis; therefore, seminiferous tubules are indirectly affected by LH secretion.

51. The answer is E. *(Speroff, ed 3. pp 285–286.)* Human chorionic gonadotropin (HCG) supports the corpus luteum of early pregnancy and can be first detected in maternal blood on about the eighth day after ovulation. This is well before a sustained rise in basal body temperature. Pelvic examination and ultrasonography do not generally detect pregnancy until about the fourth week after ovulation.

52. The answer is D. *(Speroff, ed 3. p 510.)* Severe thermal trauma to the testes, such as that caused by extremes of cold or heat, can inhibit the development of sperm. Depression in the sperm count usually appears in about 75 days, the length of time in which an immature spermatid develops into a spermatozoon. Either oligospermia or azoospermia can result.

53. The answer is B. *(Speroff, ed 3. p 233.)* The normal volume of menstrual blood loss is about 30 ml. A volume greater than 100 ml is considered abnormal. The largest part of the blood loss generally occurs on the first or second day.

54. The answer is E. *(Masters, 1966. pp 48, 56–59.)* Masters and Johnson have shown that the size of the clitoris bears no relation to increased orgasmic capacity. Similarly, the distance between the clitoris and the vaginal introitus makes little difference, because clitoral stimulation during coition is provided largely by traction on the clitoral hood via the labia minora, which are moved during penile thrusting. Direct clitoral stimulation can be achieved only by the lateral and female superior coital positions. Erection of the clitoris is likewise not related to orgasmic capacity.

55. The answer is E. *(Kase, p 1011).* The following are the failure rates with contraceptive methods: oral contraceptives 0.7 percent; IUD 1 to 3 percent; diaphragm 2 percent; spermicides 5 percent; and rhythm 15 percent. The actual effectiveness in use, however, is much lower since patients often do not use the various methods properly.

56. The answer is D. *(Speroff, ed 3. pp 75–95.)* The menstrual cycle is regulated by several hormones. FSH and estradiol stimulate the follicle in the follicular stage. LH levels rise in the late follicular phase and under the influence of estradiol surge at midcycle. LH initiates progesterone production. Progesterone induces the midcycle FSH peak, which in turn frees the oocyte from its follicular attachments. Progesterone also enhances activity of proteolytic enzymes that, along with prostaglandins, digest and rupture the follicular wall. HCG is present only if there is conception.

57. The answer is E (all). *(Kase, pp 505–506, 975.)* Vaginismus is painful spasm of the pelvic muscles and vaginal outlet and is usually psychogenic. It should be differentiated from frigidity, which implies lack of sexual desire. Treatment is primarily psychotherapeutic as organic causes are very rare.

58. The answer is E (all). *(Speroff, ed 3. pp 70–71.)* The presence of estrogen in a pubertal woman stimulates the formation of secondary sex characteristics, including development of breasts, appearance of axillary hair, production of cervical mucus, and vaginal cornification. As estrogen levels increase, menses begins and ovulation is maintained for several decades. Decreasing levels of estrogen lower the frequency of ovulation, eventually leading to the menopause.

59. The answer is E (all). *(Kase, pp 252–253.)* Delayed puberty in general is defined as absent breast budding by age 13 and delay in progression is defined as the elapsing of 5 years between onset of breast changes and the expected menarche. There are five etiologic classifications of delayed puberty. The first is constitutional delay, which is more common in girls than boys and runs in families. The second is hypergonadotropic hypogonadism, of which gonadal dysgenesis is an example. Patients with Turner syndrome are in this category. Another class is hypogonadotropic hypogonadism, which includes CNS diseases such as tumors or meningoencephalitis. The fourth class is gonadotropin deficiency, such as is seen in patients with anorexia and others with pituitary deficiency. Lastly, there is normogonadotropic hypogonadism, as in end-organ defects such as müllerian agenesis and testicular feminization.

60. The answer is C (2, 4). *(Sciarra, ed 51, vol 6, chap 47. pp 7–11.)* Vasectomy involves division of each ductus deferens via a scrotal incision. There is no demonstrable effect on androgen production, libido, or sexual performance. Granuloma formation occasionally follows, but is not a serious clinical problem. There have been some reports of antibody production to sperm after vasectomy.

61. The answer is E (all). *(Jones, ed 10. pp 804–815.)* Postmenopausal patients are subject to some unique problems. The lack of estrogen produces an atrophic vaginal mucosa with symptoms of discharge, itching, burning, and dyspareunia. The dyspareunia often leads to sexual dysfunction. Often these are accompanied by urethritis. Osteoporosis is now a well-recognized complication of the menopause. It is more common in women who are smokers. Estrogen replacement slows the rate of osteoporosis but its administration needs to be monitored for its associated risk of developing endometrial carcinoma. Estrogen replacement is now given along with progesterone. Women are also encouraged to take adequate calcium supplementation, to decrease smoking, and to exercise regularly. Many patients are depressed because of these problems and also because they do not often get the support and sympathy that they need. Many also have misconceptions about menopause because of a lack of education regarding the physiology. Supportive therapy is extremely important.

62. The answer is D (4). *(Masters, 1966. p 69.)* Masters and Johnson observed a transudate-like fluid emanating directly from the vaginal walls during sexual response. This mucoid material, which is sufficient for complete vaginal lubrication, is produced by transudation from the venous plexus surrounding the vagina and appears seconds after the initiation of sexual excitement. No activity by Skene's glands was noted, and production of cervical mucus during sexual stimulation was observed in only a very few subjects. Fluid from Bartholin's glands appears long after vaginal lubrication is well established; it may, however, make a minor contribution to lubrication in the late plateau phase.

63. The answer is E (all). *(Wilson, ed 7. pp 263–264.)* The gonadotropins (FSH and LH) are glycoproteins. In women, they stimulate the production of one or more primordial follicles and induce thecal cells in the ovary to produce estrogen. In a man who has hypopituitarism, the gonadotropins can cause production of spermatozoa and testosterone.

64. The answer is C (2, 4). *(Kase, p 337.)* Menopause is usually reached by age 50 to 52. It is preceded in some cases by vasomotor symptoms such as hot flashes and perspiration. In most women these last 1 to 2 years, but in some (as many as 25 percent) they last longer than 5 years. These vasomotor symptoms are secondary to reduced endogenous estrogen. Often FSH and LH levels rise as much as ten- to twenty-fold; they are reliable tests for menopause.

65. The answer is A (1, 2, 3). *(Masters, 1966. pp 27–37.)* The response of women to sexual stimulation is generalized and affects many different organ systems. Physiological responses include superficial and deep vasocongestion accounting for, among other things, enlargement and changes of color of extragenital and genital areas. Voluntary and involuntary myotonia, both generalized and specific, also may occur, although involuntary contractions of the rectal sphincter are usually detected only during the orgasmic phase.

66. The answer is B (1, 3). *(Speroff, ed 3. pp 9–12.)* In the luteal phase of the menstrual cycle, granulosa cells produce estrogen by way of the Δ^4-3-ketone pathway, in which progesterone is a precursor. Theca cells in the follicular phase of the menstrual cycle manufacture estrogen by the Δ^5-3β-hydroxy pathway; pregnenolone, dehydroepiandrosterone, and estradiol—but not progesterone—are essential precursors of this pathway.

67. The answer is A (1, 2, 3). *(Kase, p 1010.)* The marked effectiveness of the combined oral contraceptive pill, which contains a synthetic estrogen and a progestin, is related to its multiple antifertility actions. The primary effect is to suppress gonadotropins, thus inhibiting ovulation. The prolonged progestational effect also causes thickening of the cervical mucus and atrophic changes of the endometrium, thus impairing sperm penetrability and ovum implantation, respectively.

68. The answer is A (1, 2, 3). *(Speroff, ed 3. p 7.)* The conversion of acetate to cholesterol and, hence, to all the other steroid hormones can occur in the ovary, testis, and adrenal gland. The placenta, however, lacks the essential enzyme systems to perform this synthesis. Therefore, cholesterol, the basic building block in the synthesis of steroid hormones, must be supplied to the placenta. The fetus and the mother supply the cholesterol essential for steroidogenesis in the placenta. It has been suggested that the maternal cholesterol serves as the precursor for progesterone production, while fetal cholesterol is used for estrogen production.

69. The answer is A (1, 2, 3). *(Wilson, ed 7. pp 112–114.)* Growth hormone and chorionic somatomammotropin are polypeptide hormones composed of 191 amino-acid subunits, of which 161 are identical (the other 30 are closely related and vary by only a simple base change in the DNA template). Although the structure of human prolactin is not yet clearly established, it too is a polypeptide hormone of close to 200 subunits, many of which are in the same sequence as the other two hormones. Prolactin, growth hormone, and chorionic somatomammotropin are all able to induce hormonal changes directly in their target organs. Thyrotropin is a glycoprotein; its only physiological action is stimulation of the thyroid gland to produce another hormone, thyroxine, which is the mediator of thyroid activity.

70–74. The answers are: 70-A, 71-C, 72-B, 73-D, 74-D. *(Wilson, ed 7. pp 23, 372, 819–820, 1116.)* Testosterone reaching a target organ, such as the prostate gland, is converted to dihydrotestosterone by 5α-reductase, an enzyme in the cell wall or cell membrane. Adenylcyclase, which is an intracellular enzyme activated by the presence of LH, catalyzes the formation of cyclic AMP, which then activates other intracellular enzyme reactions. The enzyme 17β-hydroxylase is found primarily in the testis but also in the adrenal gland; it converts androstenedione to testosterone by hydroxylating the 17 position.

The conversion of cholesterol into steroid hormones begins with hydroxylation at the 30 position followed by cleavage of the six-carbon side chain (carbons 22 to 27); both reactions, which result in production of pregnenolone, are catalyzed by 20-hydroxylase (also known as cholesterol desmolase). Congenital deficiencies of this enzyme can cause the adrenal glands to fill with cholesterol and become greatly enlarged; affected infants, some of whom may be phenotypic females but genotypic males, have a poor prognosis.

Pregnancy, Lactation, and Puerperium

DIRECTIONS: Each question below contains five suggested responses. Select the **one best** response to each question.

75. The earliest diagnosis of pregnancy by a sensitive serum βHCG assay is possible

(A) 1 hour after implantation
(B) during the week before the anticipated menses
(C) the day of anticipated menses
(D) 1 week after the missed menses
(E) 10 days after the missed menses

76. During pregnancy a woman needs additional iron to satisfy the demands of the fetus, the placenta, and her own increasing hemoglobin mass. The total antepartum iron need is approximately

(A) 250 mg
(B) 800 mg
(C) 1350 mg
(D) 1900 mg
(E) none of the above

77. During pregnancy, the renal glomerular filtration rate (GFR) can increase by as much as

(A) 10 percent
(B) 25 percent
(C) 50 percent
(D) 75 percent
(E) 100 percent

78. An elevation of prolactin levels is caused by all the following physiological states EXCEPT

(A) sleep
(B) stress
(C) exercise
(D) parturition
(E) puerperium

79. Which of the following statements best characterizes the estrogen present in maternal urine?

(A) Its concentration is decreased during pregnancy
(B) It is 80 to 85 percent estriol at term
(C) It is 15 percent estrone at term
(D) Its excretion is normal at term in patients who have placental sulfatase deficiency
(E) Its excretion is unrelated to fetal adrenal or hepatic function

80. The hydronephrosis and hydroureter that develop during pregnancy resolve spontaneously by how many weeks post partum?

(A) 1 week
(B) 4 weeks
(C) 8 weeks
(D) 10 weeks
(E) 12 weeks

81. Acute puerperal mastitis is characterized by all the following statements EXCEPT

(A) the initial treatment is antibiotics
(B) the source of the infection is usually the infant's nose and throat
(C) frank abscesses may develop and require drainage
(D) the most common offending organism is *Escherichia coli*
(E) the symptoms include chills, fever, and tachycardia

82. The maximum amniotic fluid volume is usually reached at what gestational age?

(A) 32 to 34 weeks
(B) 34 to 36 weeks
(C) 36 to 38 weeks
(D) 38 to 40 weeks
(E) 40 to 42 weeks

83. As pregnancy progresses, which of the following hematological changes occurs?

(A) Plasma volume increases proportionally more than red-cell volume
(B) Red-cell volume increases proportionally more than plasma volume
(C) Plasma volume increases and red-cell volume remains constant
(D) Red-cell volume decreases and plasma volume remains constant
(E) Neither plasma volume nor red-cell volume changes

84. Maternal mortality refers to the number of maternal deaths that occur as the result of the reproductive process per

(A) 1000 births
(B) 10,000 births
(C) 100,000 births
(D) 10,000 live births
(E) 100,000 live births

85. A 23-year-old woman (gravida 2, para 2) calls her physician 7 days post partum because she is concerned that she is still bleeding from the vagina. It would be appropriate to tell this woman that it is normal for bloody lochia to last up to

(A) 2 days
(B) 5 days
(C) 8 days
(D) 11 days
(E) 14 days

DIRECTIONS: Each question below contains four suggested responses of which **one or more** is correct. Select

A	if	**1, 2, and 3**	are correct
B	if	**1 and 3**	are correct
C	if	**2 and 4**	are correct
D	if	**4**	is correct
E	if	**1, 2, 3, and 4**	are correct

86. Changes in the respiratory system during pregnancy include

(1) increased tidal volume
(2) decreased residual volume
(3) increased respiratory minute volume
(4) increased respiratory rate

87. Which of the following physiological changes can occur during a normal pregnancy?

(1) Decrease in fasting blood β-hydroxybutyric acid
(2) Increase in postprandial blood glucose
(3) Increase in fasting blood glucose
(4) Increase in postprandial insulin

88. Which of the following thyroxine-related changes can occur during pregnancy?

(1) Increase of total serum thyroxine
(2) Increase of free thyroxine
(3) Increase of thyroxine-binding globulin
(4) Decrease of thyroid-stimulating hormone

89. Which of the following laboratory values can be expected to increase during pregnancy?

(1) Serum albumin
(2) Plasma fibrinogen
(3) Blood urea nitrogen
(4) Erythrocyte sedimentation rate

90. Insulin secretion in pregnancy is increased by

(1) progesterone
(2) estrogen
(3) growth hormone
(4) human chorionic somatomammotropin

91. Ureteral dilatation during pregnancy is caused by which of the following?

(1) Uterine pressure at the pelvic brim
(2) Pressure from the dilated right ovarian vein
(3) Progesterone effect
(4) The increased glomerular filtration rate

A	B	C	D	E
1,2,3 only	1,3 only	2,4 only	4 only	All are correct

92. True statements about breast cancer include that it

(1) cannot be safely diagnosed by mammogram in pregnancy
(2) may mimic benign mastitis in pregnancy
(3) is a contraindication for future pregnancy
(4) should be treated the same in the first and second trimester of pregnancy as in the nonpregnant patient

93. Correct statements regarding lactation following delivery include that

(1) menstruation may resume by 6 to 8 weeks in most nonlactating women
(2) approximately one third of lactating women will resume menses by 3 months
(3) ovulation may occur within 6 weeks in lactating women
(4) women treated with bromocryptine for lactation suppression may ovulate by the second postpartum week

94. In the mother, suckling leads to which of the following responses?

(1) Release of oxytocin
(2) Decrease of prolactin inhibitory factor
(3) Decrease of hypothalamic dopamine
(4) Increase of luteinizing-hormone releasing factor

95. True statements regarding postpartum depression include which of the following?

(1) A history of depression is a risk factor for developing postpartum depression
(2) Prenatal preventive intervention for patients at high risk for postpartum depression is best managed alone by a mental health professional
(3) Postpartum depression is a self-limiting process that lasts for a maximum of 3 months
(4) About 10 to 12 percent of women develop postpartum depression

96. An inability to void in the puerperium may be due to

(1) a vulvar hematoma
(2) urethral trauma
(3) use of general anesthesia
(4) infusion of oxytocin after delivery

Pregnancy, Lactation, and Puerperium

Answers

75. The answer is B. *(Danforth, ed 4. p 343. Speroff, ed 3. p 286.)* Sensitive assays use radioimmunoassay and employ antibodies specific to the β subunit of HCG. Many assays use a cutoff point of approximately 35 mIU/ml. βHCG can be demonstrated on the ninth day past the midcycle gonadotropin surge, which corresponds to 8 days past ovulation and 1 day following implantation.

76. The answer is B. *(Pritchard, ed 17. pp 251–253.)* The fetus and placenta contain approximately 300 mg of elemental iron at birth. In addition, the maternal increase in hemoglobin mass accounts for about 500 mg of elemental iron. Thus, the total antepartum iron requirement is 800 mg. Most of this iron is needed during the second half of pregnancy, at an approximate rate of 5.7 mg daily during the last 140 days. However, because about 1 mg of iron is excreted daily, the total daily iron need is almost 7 mg during the second half of pregnancy. Most women of childbearing age cannot mobilize this much iron, and supplemental iron must be given to prevent iron deficiency. The usual iron supplement, ferrous sulfate, contains 20 percent elemental iron. Thus, a 325-mg tablet contains about 65 mg of elemental iron, of which 10 to 20 percent will be absorbed. Most prenatal vitamins contain 60 or 65 mg of iron, and these should be adequate for a healthy pregnant woman. If iron stores have been depleted by poor dietary habits, recent childbirth, or other causes, however, additional iron supplementation may be necessary.

77. The answer is C. *(Pritchard, ed 17. p 197.)* The glomerular filtration rate (GFR) increases early in pregnancy—by as much as 50 percent by the beginning of the second trimester. The elevated GFR persists to term. The precise mechanism has not been identified.

78. The answer is E. *(Wilson, ed 7. pp 607–608.)* Prolactin is released episodically in humans, with the highest levels being recorded during the nocturnal sleeping hours and the lowest levels during the waking hours of 10 AM to 12 AM. Several other physiological stimuli, such as the stress of anesthesia, surgery, and exercise, have been shown to cause a rise in prolactin levels. In women, prolactin levels start to rise during the first trimester of pregnancy to a concentration ten times greater than that of the nonpregnant state. In the puerperium, prolactin levels decrease, reaching the normal range by the second or third week after delivery.

79. The answer is B. *(Aladjem, ed 2. pp 262–266.)* Total urinary estrogen at term is markedly elevated when compared with that of a nonpregnant woman. Estriol constitutes 80 to 85 percent of this urinary estrogen; its precursors are derived from the fetal liver and adrenal glands. When placental sulfatase activity is diminished, urinary excretion of estriol markedly decreases.

80. The answer is C. *(Pritchard, ed 17. p 200.)* After delivery, resolution of hydronephrosis and hydroureter is complete by 6 to 8 weeks. There is no permanent impairment. Extreme caution must be exercised in the interpretation of radiographic studies in the postpartum period so as not to inappropriately diagnose pathology that is really just a physiologic alteration.

81. The answer is D. *(Pritchard, ed 17. pp 740–741.)* Puerperal mastitis may be subacute but is often characterized by chills, fever, and tachycardia. If undiagnosed it may progress to suppurative mastitis with abscess formation that requires drainage. The most common offending organism is *Staphylococcus aureus*, which probably is transmitted from the infant's nose and throat. This in turn is most likely acquired from personnel in the nursery. At times, epidemics of suppurative mastitis have developed. A penicillinase-resistant antibiotic is the initial treatment of choice.

82. The answer is C. *(Pritchard, ed 17. pp 169–170, 462–463.)* The maximum amniotic fluid volume of 1 L is reached at 36 to 38 weeks gestation. A decrease in volume is usually noted as term approaches, and in the postterm pregnancy clinically apparent oligohydramnios may develop. Oligohydramnios may also occur in association with fetal renal agenesis (Potter syndrome) and in some cases of intrauterine growth retardation.

83. The answer is A. *(Danforth, ed 4. p 331.)* During pregnancy, the plasma volume increases by about 48 percent and the red-cell volume increases by about 30 percent. The rapid increase in the plasma volume occurs during early pregnancy, while the red-cell volume rises more rapidly after the first trimester of pregnancy. As a result, the hematocrit during the first trimester and most of the second trimester of pregnancy could be much lower than normal. The reduction in hematocrit constitutes the "physiological anemia" of pregnancy.

84. The answer is E. *(Pritchard, ed 17. pp 2–4.)* Maternal mortality is calculated per 100,000 live births. Although there have been marked advances in prenatal care associated with a declining maternal mortality over the past 25 years, there still exist subgroups of the female population at much higher risk. These include black women (apparently because of social and economic conditions), women of high parity, and the older gravida. About 50 percent of maternal deaths in the United States are caused by hemorrhage, hypertension, or infection.

85. The answer is E. *(Pritchard, ed 17. pp 373–374.)* Bloody lochia can persist for up to 2 weeks without indicating an underlying pathology; however, if bleeding continues beyond 2 weeks, it may indicate placental site subinvolution, retention of small placental fragments, or both. At this point, appropriate diagnostic and thera-peutic measures should be initiated. The physician should first estimate the blood loss and then perform a pelvic examination in search of uterine subinvolution or tenderness. Excessive bleeding or tenderness should lead the physician to suspect retained placental fragments or endometritis. A larger-than-expected but otherwise asymptomatic uterus supports the diagnosis of subinvolution.

86. The answer is A (1, 2, 3). *(Sciarra, ed 51, vol 2, chap 26. p 5.)* Progesterone is thought to result in gradually increasing tidal volume (volume of air moved) to 30 to 40 percent above baseline at term. Although respiratory rate remains un-changed, the increased respiratory minute volume causes a decrease in CO_2 in the alveoli and blood resulting in the "hyperventilation" of the pregnancy.

87. The answer is C (2, 4). *(Burrow, ed 2. pp 36–39.)* During pregnancy fasting blood glucose levels generally decrease, probably because the fetus, needing tre-mendous amounts of glucose, takes glucose at the expense of the mother. In addition, the maternal response to fasting is accentuated by pregnancy and results in exag-gerated starvation ketosis and increased fasting levels of β-hydroxybutyric acid (a ketone body). For a number of reasons, insulin is less effective during pregnancy in diminishing blood glucose. Postprandial blood glucose therefore tends to be higher than in the nonpregnant state, and results of a glucose tolerance test must be inter-preted differently. To offset anti-insulin effects, insulin production is augmented during the normal pregnancy, and postprandial insulin levels are increased.

88. The answer is B (1, 3). *(Burrow, ed 2. pp 188–191.)* Probably because of increased estrogen levels, pregnancy is associated with an increase in the amounts of many proteins in the serum, among them thyroxine-binding globulin. In order to maintain normal levels of free thyroxine and triiodothyronine, more total thyroxine must be produced to tie up some of the excess binding sites on the carrier protein. Therefore, the total serum thyroxine concentration increases while the level of free thyroxine stays constant. Thyroid-stimulating hormone (TSH) levels are slightly increased during early pregnancy but by term are back in the normal range, as measured by radioimmunoassay. There are some data to suggest that TSH-like activity also is increased in pregnancy, possibly owing to a placental factor, either human chorionic gonadotropin or human chorionic thyrotropin. This explanation applies especially to pregnancies complicated by trophoblastic disease.

89. The answer is C (2, 4). *(Pritchard, ed 17. pp 188–191.)* Plasma fibrinogen levels increase by about 50 percent during pregnancy. This rise is thought to be at least partially responsible for the great increase in the erythrocyte sedimentation rate. The elevated sedimentation rate is consequently almost useless as a significant laboratory value in pregnant women. Serum albumin decreases by about 30 percent during normal pregnancy. Blood urea nitrogen (BUN) decreases markedly during pregnancy; in fact, BUN values falling in the middle of the normal range for non-pregnant women (i.e., around 10 mg/100 ml) may signal significant impairment of renal function in pregnant women.

90. The answer is D (4). *(Burrow, ed 2. pp 40–41.)* The tendency for pregnancy to be diabetogenic is thought to be due mainly to the anti-insulin effects of many of the hormones secreted by the placenta as well as to the possible effect of insulin receptors on the placenta itself. Human chorionic somatomammotropin (also known as human placental lactogen) is present in large amounts in the maternal circulation during the third trimester. Its lipolytic and other actions inhibit glucose uptake and manufacture and therefore stimulate insulin production to rise. Levels of pituitary growth hormone are decreased, especially during late pregnancy, and probably have little to do with increased insulin needs. Estrogen and probably progesterone, both of which are present in increased amounts during pregnancy, probably act as peripheral insulin antagonists and therefore would lead to decreased insulin utilization.

91. The answer is A (1, 2, 3). *(Pritchard, ed 17. pp 198–199.)* One of the common areas of ureteral compression is at the pelvic brim. As the uterus rises out of the pelvis it compresses the ureters at the pelvic brim. The right ureter seems to be dilated more than the left ureter and it is thought that the dilated right ovarian vein contributes to the pressure on the right. Progesterone is a smooth muscle relaxant and it may contribute to the presence of the hydroureters. An increased glomerular filtration rate would not cause the ureters to dilate.

92. The answer is C (2, 4). *(Burrow, ed 2. pp 521–523.)* The diagnosis of breast cancer in pregnancy is more difficult because of the enlargement and hypervascularity of tissue. If associated with lymphatic obstruction, cancer may mimic benign mastitis. Although mammography should not be used for routine screening, it is the diagnostic imaging of choice and can be performed safely with abdominal shielding. All suspicious masses by palpation and either mammography or thermography should have excisional biopsy regardless of pregnancy and, depending on results, definitive surgery. Therapeutic abortion is considered only to facilitate treatment of metastatic disease; however, chemotherapy has not been implicated in malformations. Risk of disease recurrence has not been shown to increase with future pregnancies.

93. The answer is E (all). *(Pritchard ed 17. p 376. Speroff, ed 3. p 250.)* Various studies have confirmed all the statements presented in the question. It is thus vital to warn all postpartum women that they can become pregnant even within the first postpartum month, whether or not they are breast-feeding. At some centers, patients considered at high risk for pregnancy will be started on birth control pills upon discharge from the hospital.

94. The answer is A (1, 2, 3). *(Speroff, ed 3. pp 246–250.)* The normal sequence of events triggered by suckling is as follows: through a response of the central nervous system, dopamine is decreased in the hypothalamus. Dopamine suppression decreases production of prolactin inhibitory factor (PIF), which normally travels through a portal system to the pituitary gland; because PIF production is decreased, production of prolactin by the pituitary is increased. At this time, the pituitary also releases oxytocin, which causes milk to be expressed from the alveoli into the lactiferous ducts. Suckling suppresses the production of luteinizing-hormone (LH) releasing factor and, as a result, acts as a mild contraceptive (the midcycle LH surge does not occur).

95. The answer is D (4). *(Pritchard, ed 17. p 375.)* Patients at high risk for postpartum depression often have histories of depression or postpartum depression. They are more likely to be primiparous or older; they may have had a long interval between pregnancies, an unplanned pregnancy, or be without a supportive partner. Prenatal intervention must include the obstetric team with family or peer support when possible. Postpartum depression is variable in duration, but occasionally will not resolve without hospitalization, therapy, or medication.

96. The answer is E (all). *(Pritchard, ed 17. p 739.)* An inability to void often leads to the diagnosis of a vulvar hematoma. It is often large enough to apply pressure on the urethra. Pain from urethral lacerations is another reason women have difficulty voiding after delivery. Both general anesthesia, which temporarily disturbs neural control of the bladder, and oxytocin, which has an antidiuretic effect, can lead to an overdistended bladder and an inability to void. In this case an indwelling catheter should be inserted and left in for at least 24 hours to allow recovery of normal bladder tone and sensation.

PRIMARY CARE

History, Physical Examination, and Diagnostic Procedures

DIRECTIONS: Each question below contains five suggested responses. Select the **one best** response to each question.

97. False positive Venereal Disease Research Laboratories (VDRL) tests have been associated with all the following EXCEPT

(A) narcotic addiction
(B) atypical pneumonias
(C) old age
(D) diabetes mellitus
(E) leprosy

98. Routine pelvic examination reveals that a 21-year-old woman has a hooded cervix. This finding is most frequently associated with

(A) pregnancy
(B) traumatic abortion
(C) in utero drug exposure
(D) a prior Shirodkar procedure
(E) a herpesvirus infection

99. All the following statements concerning a hysterosalpingogram test for fallopian-tube patency are true EXCEPT that

(A) the contrast medium used may be either oil- or water-soluble
(B) salpingitis isthmica nodosa may be diagnosed with this procedure
(C) abnormalities of the uterine cavity may be diagnosed with this procedure
(D) less than 3 ml of contrast medium should be used to avoid spill from the tubes into the peritoneal cavity
(E) the test may have a therapeutic effect on infertility

100. All the following tests would be helpful in the diagnosis of an ectopic pregnancy EXCEPT

(A) a pregnancy test
(B) culdocentesis
(C) an abdominal flat plate
(D) ultrasound
(E) a pelvic examination

101. A 19-year-old nulliparous woman is given a VDRL test, which is positive at a dilution of 1:4. The diagnostic measure that now should be ordered is a

(A) Wassermann-type test
(B) rapid plasma reagin (RPR) card test
(C) FTA-ABS test
(D) lumbar puncture and VDRL titer of cerebrospinal fluid
(E) thorough pelvic examination

102. On a routine examination, a pelvic mass is found in a 40-year-old woman. Which test would be LEAST helpful in evaluating the mass?

(A) Pelvic ultrasound
(B) Pap smear
(C) CT scan of pelvis
(D) Laparoscopy
(E) Abdominal flat plate

103. To assess the condition of the fetus in a woman who is sensitized against the Rh antigen, amniotic fluid would be withdrawn for which of the following tests?

(A) Antibody titer
(B) L/S ratio
(C) Kleinhauer-Betke test
(D) Spectrophotometric analysis (Δ OD_{450})
(E) Gram stain

DIRECTIONS: Each question below contains four suggested responses of which **one or more** is correct. Select

A	if	**1, 2, and 3**	are correct
B	if	**1 and 3**	are correct
C	if	**2 and 4**	are correct
D	if	**4**	is correct
E	if	**1, 2, 3, and 4**	are correct

104. A direct Coombs' test is correctly described by which of the following statements?

(1) It can be useful in analyzing the cord blood of babies at risk for Rh disease
(2) It involves an antiglobulin reagent made by immunizing rabbits to human immunoglobulin
(3) It cannot be used to quantify the amount of an antibody present
(4) It can be performed on the sera of pregnant RH-negative women to determine the degree of their Rh sensitization

105. A patient complains of a vaginal discharge. Which of the following tests would be helpful in deciding on her therapy?

(1) Fungal culture
(2) Pelvic examination
(3) Saline suspension for microscopic examination
(4) Noting the color of the discharge

106. As a description of a woman's obstetrical history, the digits 7-2-1-6 indicate that she has

(1) given birth to six term infants
(2) had two premature deliveries
(3) been pregnant seven times
(4) had one abortion

107. A 35-year-old woman who has had two normal children presents with the complaint of amenorrhea for 2 months. Which of the following tests should be considered?

(1) Endometrial biopsy
(2) Thyroid function tests
(3) Pregnancy test
(4) LH, FSH levels

108. Pelvic examination is an important means of diagnosing ovarian malignancies. An ovarian tumor has an increased likelihood of being malignant if examination reveals that it is

(1) mobile
(2) bilateral
(3) cystic
(4) greater than 10 cm in diameter

DIRECTIONS: Each group of questions below consists of lettered headings followed by a set of numbered items. For each numbered item select the **one** lettered heading with which it is **most** closely associated. Each lettered heading may be used **once, more than once, or not at all.**

Questions 109–111

For each of the sets of signs below, select the most likely diagnosis.

(A) Turner syndrome
(B) Pituitary adenoma
(C) Testicular feminization
(D) Swyer syndrome
(E) None of the above

109. 1° amenorrhea, infantile female sexual development

110. 1° amenorrhea, short stature, shield chest

111. 1° amenorrhea, normal breast development, absent pubic and axillary hair

Questions 112–115

For each of the patients below, select the ultrasonic finding of most concern.

(A) Fetal ascites
(B) Spinal defects
(C) Twins
(D) Short femur length
(E) Malposition of the placenta

112. A patient is 20 weeks pregnant by her last menstrual period but measures 30 cm in fundal height

113. A patient is 24 weeks pregnant and is seen after an episode of heavy bleeding per vagina

114. A patient is Rh sensitized and has had a previous stillbirth

115. A patient is referred for an ultrasound because of two elevated serum alpha-fetoprotein levels

Questions 116–118

For each of the descriptions below, select the pelvic type with which it is most likely to be associated.

(A) Anthropoid
(B) Android
(C) Gynecoid
(D) Platypelloid
(E) None of the above

116. Examination of the pelvis reveals prominent ischial spines, a narrow subpubic arch, a narrow high-arched sacrosciatic notch, a straight sacrum, and a shortened posterior sagittal diameter

117. Examination of the pelvis reveals a wide subpubic arch, a curved sacrum, and a shortened anteroposterior diameter

118. Examination of the pelvis reveals a lengthened anteroposterior diameter, a large sacrosciatic notch, prominent ischial spines, and a straight, posteriorly inclined sacrum

History, Physical Examination, and Diagnostic Procedures

Answers

97. The answer is D. *(Blaustein, ed 2. p 20.)* The VDRL is a serological test widely used to screen for syphilis. False positives appear in approximately 3 to 4 percent of all VDRL tests performed. If a false positive occurs, a physician first should ensure that the result is not due to technical error and second should consider the various entities that result in false positives at the following rates: leprosy (8 to 28 percent), smallpox vaccination (1 to 2 percent), narcotic addiction (20 to 25 percent), and old age (10 percent of patients between 70 and 80 years of age). Atypical pneumonias have also resulted in false positives. The fluorescent treponemal antibody absorption (FTA-ABS) test, which is quite specific, should be used with a borderline or suspected false positive VDRL test.

98. The answer is C. *(Danforth, ed 4. p 895.)* A hooded cervix, a "cockscomb" cervix, and cervical pseudopolyps are common structural changes associated with in utero exposure to diethylstilbestrol or chemically related nonsteroidal estrogens. Cervical erosions are almost always found in affected individuals, and vaginal adenosis is frequently present. Carcinomas of the vagina are much less frequently diagnosed.

99. The answer is D. *(Speroff, ed 3. pp 475–476.)* A hysterosalpingogram is a procedure in which 3 to 6 ml of either an oil- or water-soluble contrast medium is injected through the cervix in order to outline the uterine cavity and fallopian tubes. Spill of contrast medium into the peritoneal cavity proves patency of the uterine cavity and fallopian tubes. By outlining the cavity, abnormalities such as bicornuate uterus, uterine polyps, submucous myomas, salpingitis isthmica nodosum, and hydrosalpinx can be identified. Some controlled studies have shown a therapeutic effect resulting in an increased rate of pregnancy in infertility patients.

100. The answer is C. *(Kase, pp 541–542.)* A positive pregnancy test would confirm the presence of a pregnancy. The culdocentesis is useful in finding non-clotting blood when there is intraperitoneal bleeding from an ectopic pregnancy. Ultrasound can rule out an ectopic pregnancy by finding an intrauterine pregnancy. A pelvic examination could detect an adnexal mass. The findings on an abdominal flat plate would be nonspecific in an ectopic pregnancy.

101. The answer is C. *(Wynn, ed 3. pp 184–185.)* Because a positive VDRL test may either indicate the presence of syphilis or be a biological false positive, a specific treponemal test, such as the FTA-ABS test, is needed to discriminate false positives from true infection. The rapid plasma reagin (RPR) card test and Wassermann-type tests, such as the Kolmer test, are nontreponemal tests and therefore are no more specific than the VDRL test. A lumbar puncture would not be indicated at this point. A pelvic examination may be of little diagnostic use, because chancres often disappear before a VDRL test becomes positive.

102. The answer is B. *(Kase, p 560.)* The Pap smear evaluates cervical cytology only and gives no information on the ovaries or uterus. Pelvic ultrasound and CT scan can identify masses in the ovary or uterus, provide dimensions, and give some insight into the density and character of the tissue. Laparoscopy is helpful in allowing direct visualization of the pelvic organs. The abdominal flat plate can identify calcifications in such lesions as the benign teratoma. It can also confirm the presence of a mass and give an estimate of its dimensions.

103. The answer is D. *(Pritchard, ed 17. pp 773–778.)* The amniotic fluid is analyzed spectrophotometrically for a change in the optical density at 450 μm wavelength. The change is due to bilirubin in the fluid that comes from fetal hemolysis. According to Liley, who constructed a graph for predicting severity of disease, the higher the optical density, the more severe the hemolysis. The antibody titer is done on maternal serum and is not helpful in a woman who is already sensitized. The L/S ratio measures fetal lung maturity. The Kleinhauer-Betke test looks for fetal red blood cells and does not give any information on the status of an Rh-sensitized pregnancy since it is not a fetal intraamniotic bleed that we are concerned about. A Gram stain looks for bacteria and not bilirubin.

104. The answer is A (1, 2, 3). *(Queenan, ed 2. pp 14–15.)* The direct Coombs' test, which uses human antiglobulin derived from immunized rabbits, is performed on blood cells to determine if they are coated with antibody. A direct Coombs' test, therefore, can be useful in analyzing the cord blood of an infant who is at risk for Rh disease. Quantification of antibody titers can be achieved by doing serial dilutions of the indirect Coombs' test, which analyzes serum.

105. The answer is B (1, 3). *(Kase, pp 595–600.)* Fungal cultures can confirm and identify the type of fungal organism. A wet smear for microscopic examination can miss a large percentage of fungal infections. Saline suspension is used to look for *Trichomonas vaginalis* organisms and for clue cells that are associated with *Gardnerella vaginalis* vaginitis. A pelvic examination is not helpful and most discharges are of a white or yellowish color, so these would not help to identify the etiologic organism.

106. The answer is C (2, 4). *(Pritchard, ed 17. pp 245–246.)* Describing an obstetrical history by the four-digit system is more comprehensive than merely indicating gravidity and parity. The first digit of the four indicates the number of term infants delivered; the second, the number of premature infants delivered; the third, the number of abortions; and the fourth, the number of children now alive. A woman described as 7-2-1-6, therefore, has had seven term deliveries, two premature deliveries, and one abortion; six of her children currently are alive.

107. The answer is E (all). *(Kase, pp 271–277.)* This patient has secondary amenorrhea, which rules out abnormalities associated with primary amenorrhea such as chromosomal abnormalities and outflow tract abnormalities. The most common reason for amenorrhea in a woman of reproductive age is pregnancy. Other possibilities include chronic endometritis or scarring of the endometrium (Asherman syndrome), hypothyroidism, and premature ovarian failure. In addition emotional stress, extreme weight loss, and adrenal cortical insufficiency can bring about secondary amenorrhea.

108. The answer is C (2, 4). *(Wynn, ed 3. p 267.)* Unilateral, cystic, mobile, and small (less than 10 cm) adnexal masses tend to be benign neoplasms. Masses that are bilateral, solid, fixed, and large, on the other hand, more characteristically are malignant and require prompt diagnostic evaluation and treatment. Ascites also is frequently associated with ovarian malignancies.

109–111. The answers are: 109-D, 110-A, 111-C. *(Speroff, ed 3. pp 156–164, 173, 177.)* After obtaining a history and performing a physical examination, other testing may be helpful in diagnosing causes of amenorrhea. An abnormal karyotype will be seen with Turner syndrome (45,X) testicular feminization (46,XY), and Swyer syndrome (46,XY). Testosterone levels will distinguish between the latter two conditions. Such diagnosis is important because the streak gonads in Swyer syndrome have high potential for transformation and should be removed as soon as diagnosis is made, whereas those in testicular feminization can be retained until after puberty.

112–115. The answers are: 112-C, 113-E, 114-A, 115-B. *(Pritchard, ed 17. pp 277–278, 409–411, 511, 776.)* A patient whose size is greater than her dates should always have an ultrasound examination to rule out multiple gestations.

Any bleeding during pregnancy should be investigated—especially heavy bleeding after the first trimester. The conditions that we are especially concerned about are placenta previa and low lying placentas.

Rh sensitization that causes severe fetal anemia could lead to hydrops fetalis, a severe subcutaneous edema and effusion into serous cavities, such as into the abdominal cavity, that causes ascites. Portal hypertension, severe hypoalbuminemia, and heart failure contribute to the ascites.

Assuming that the dates are correct, the most common reason for an elevated maternal serum alpha-fetoprotein level is an open neural tube defect such as open spina bifida or anencephaly. At the same time that an ultrasound examination is obtained, an amniocentesis is also done to look for elevated levels in amniotic fluid.

116–118. The answers are: 116-B, 117-D, 118-A. *(Pritchard, ed 17. pp 221–235.)* The four general pelvic configurations, named here according to the widely used Caldwell-Moloy classification, may be important indicators of potential problems during labor and delivery. The gynecoid pelvis, the most common type, is generally round, with the transverse diameter being the same as or slightly greater than the anteroposterior diameter.

The anthropoid pelvis is essentially oblong, with the anteroposterior diameter being much greater than the transverse diameter. It is thus a deep, narrow pelvis; characteristically, the ischial spines are prominent and the sacrum is inclined posteriorly.

The android pelvis is often described as triangular. The anterior pelvis is narrowed, with a narrow subpubic angle; but, unlike the anthropoid pelvis, the posterior pelvis is short, with a small posterior sagittal diameter. The spines are prominent in the android pelvis, and the sacrum is straight. Unless it is unusually large, this type of pelvis offers a poor prognosis for delivery.

The rarest pelvic type is the platypelloid ("flat") pelvis. Here the anteroposterior diameter is quite short and the transverse diameter is wide. The subpubic angle is wide and the ischial spines are not prominent. This type of pelvis may cause the vertex to stay in the occiput transverse position until delivery.

Clinical, Behavioral, Medical, and Legal Problems

DIRECTIONS: Each question below contains five suggested responses. Select the **one best** response to each question.

119. The management of girls who have idiopathic precocious puberty includes

(A) progestin therapy
(B) estrogen therapy
(C) androgen therapy
(D) pelvic irradiation
(E) laparoscopy

120. A 22-year-old woman, gravida 3, para 2 (one abortion), is brought to the hospital because she says she has been raped by a 35-year-old man whom she knows to have had a vasectomy 2 years ago. Both individuals have an A-positive blood type. Which of the following would be most useful to her in the prosecution of this case?

(A) Accurate description of the introitus
(B) Smear for sperm from the cervix
(C) Vaginal washings for acid phosphatase
(D) Specific typing of vaginal washings
(E) Examination of her pubic hair

121. In the experience of Masters and Johnson and other sex therapists, the sexual dysfunction having the lowest cure rate is

(A) premature ejaculation
(B) vaginismus
(C) primary impotence
(D) secondary impotence
(E) female orgasmic dysfunction

122. Of the following, the most significant risk factor for developing breast cancer is

(A) the presence of sclerosing adenosis
(B) nulliparity
(C) atypical lobular hyperplasia
(D) atypical ductal hyperplasia
(E) menarche before age 12

123. Which of the following statements about breast cancer is true?

(A) It is the most common cause of a bloody nipple discharge
(B) It is often preceded by breast cysts
(C) If malignant, well over 50 percent are infiltrating duct carcinomas
(D) Most breast masses are initially found by the physician
(E) A bloody nipple discharge is usually the initial symptom

124. The most common cause of precocious puberty in girls is

(A) idiopathic
(B) gonadal tumors
(C) Albright syndrome
(D) hypothyroidism
(E) central nervous system tumors

125. High risk factors for development of adverse psychological responses to gynecologic surgery include all the following EXCEPT

(A) age less than 35
(B) nulliparity
(C) prior psychiatric history
(D) absence of proven surgical pathology
(E) over 12 years of formal education

126. A 46-year-old woman presents with depression, urinary urgency, night sweats, and headaches. On examination she is found to be anovulatory. The most likely diagnosis is

(A) psychosomatic disorder
(B) manic depression
(C) urinary tract infection
(D) tuberculosis with renal involvement
(E) menopause

127. True statements about lesbians include that

(A) most lesbians would like to have children
(B) their behavior is associated with an abnormal hormonal state
(C) they have been found to have different personality characteristics from other women
(D) most lesbians are quite open in telling their physicians about their situation
(E) lesbians who do not inform their physicians of their situation refrain out of fear of jeopardizing their medical care

128. Which of the following is the correct chronological order of stages of puberty?

(A) Accelerated growth spurt, breast budding, pubarche, menarche
(B) Accelerated growth spurt, pubarche, breast budding, menarche
(C) Breast budding, accelerated growth spurt, pubarche, menarche
(D) Breast budding, pubarche, menarche, accelerated growth spurt
(E) Pubarche, breast budding, accelerated growth spurt, menarche

DIRECTIONS: Each question below contains four suggested responses of which **one or more** is correct. Select

A	if	**1, 2, and 3**	are correct
B	if	**1 and 3**	are correct
C	if	**2 and 4**	are correct
D	if	**4**	is correct
E	if	**1, 2, 3, and 4**	are correct

129. True statements about the creation of the patient-physician relationship include which of the following?

(1) The patient-physician relationship is considered a contract
(2) The patient has the right to accept or reject the physician's proposed service as part of the contract
(3) A consent is not considered valid unless the patient comprehends the involved treatment and its ramifications
(4) If the physician begins treatment, he or she is considered to be involved in the contract

130. Endocrine-related causes of short stature in young women include

(1) hypothyroidism
(2) adrenal hyperplasia
(3) Cushing's disease
(4) Turner syndrome

131. Estrogen administration is considered advantageous in the treatment of perimenopausal women who have

(1) emotional reactions
(2) vasomotor reactions
(3) osteoporosis
(4) epithelial atrophy

132. Delayed puberty should be suspected if

(1) breast budding is still absent by age 13
(2) 5 years have elapsed between the onset of breast budding and the expected menarche
(3) menarche is delayed beyond 16 years of age
(4) FSH is greater than 40 mIU/ml at age 16

133. Primary orgasmic dysfunction in women can be described by which of the following statements?

(1) It can stem from dissatisfaction with a partner's behavior patterns
(2) The influence of orthodox religious beliefs is still of major etiological significance
(3) It can be exacerbated if a partner suffers from premature ejaculation
(4) A woman affected by it has never in her life achieved orgasm

134. A woman may experience orgasm by

(1) clitoral stimulation
(2) dreams
(3) vaginal stimulation
(4) extragenital stimulation

135. True statements about postpartum depression include which of the following?

(1) It has a recurrence rate as high as 50 percent
(2) It most commonly develops 4 to 8 months after delivery
(3) It is more likely in women with a prior psychological history
(4) It is to a large extent related to hormonal changes around the time of delivery

136. True statements regarding rape by a known (versus an unknown) assailant include which of the following?

(1) Long-term sexual difficulties arise more frequently when a patient is the victim of rape by an unknown assailant
(2) Rape by a stranger is far more likely to be reported than rape by a known assailant
(3) Sexual adjustment is easier after rape by a known assailant
(4) Many women with sexual dysfunction may be sufferers of "silent rape" syndrome

137. Dyspareunia may be the result of

(1) psychological etiology
(2) organic causes
(3) birth-control pills with high estrogen content
(4) intrauterine devices

138. Treatment for dysfunctional uterine bleeding may include

(1) progestin therapy
(2) combined birth-control therapy
(3) estrogen therapy
(4) antiprostaglandin therapy

139. The use of estrogen replacement therapy may be hazardous, if not expressly contraindicated, for women who have

(1) impaired hepatic function
(2) thromboembolic disorders
(3) estrogen-dependent tumors
(4) a mother or sister with osteoporosis

140. True statements regarding psychological symptoms of the climacteric include which of the following?

(1) They include insomnia, irritability, frustration, and malaise
(2) They are due to a drop in estrogen levels
(3) They are the result of interaction of many factors
(4) They are a reaction to the cessation of menstrual flow

DIRECTIONS: The group of questions below consists of lettered headings followed by a set of numbered items. For each numbered item select the **one** lettered heading with which it is **most** closely associated. Each lettered heading may be used **once, more than once, or not at all.**

Questions 141–145

For each of the circumstances of death that might occur in a patient with generalized carcinomatosis, select the correct term used to describe the occurrence.

(A) Natural death
(B) Passive euthanasia
(C) Active euthanasia
(D) Facilitated suicide
(E) Suicide

141. Coincidental myocardial infarction with failure of resuscitative efforts

142. Overdose of barbiturates procured by the patient and administered by the patient without the physician's consent

143. Overdose of barbiturates procured by the physician and administered by the patient with the physician's and patient's consent

144. Overdose of barbiturates procured by the physician and administered by the physician with the physician's and patient's consent

145. Myocardial infarction with no attempt at resuscitative efforts

Clinical, Behavioral, Medical, and Legal Problems

Answers

119. The answer is A. *(Speroff, ed 3. pp. 375–376.)* Progestin therapy is the treatment of choice for girls who have idiopathic precocious puberty. Although progestins cannot cause pubic hair to disappear, they can stop future growth, arrest breast development, and, most important, cause bone growth to decelerate, thus preventing early epiphyseal closure. Estrogen treatment is contraindicated because it can only exacerbate symptoms of precocity and result in short stature. Laparoscopy is not indicated because most causes of precocious puberty can eventually be determined without surgery.

120. The answer is C. *(American College of Obstetricians and Gynecologists, ACOG Tech Bull 14: July, 1972.)* Although all the procedures mentioned in the question can be helpful in establishing a case of rape in most situations, the expected lack of sperm and the matching blood types in the situation presented would limit their value in this case. Only the finding of 50 units/ml or more of acid phosphatase in this woman's vagina could be taken as evidence of ejaculation. Her introitus probably would not be injured because of her parity. Foreign pubic hair might only indicate close contact.

121. The answer is C. *(Masters, 1970, p 367.)* In a 5-year follow-up study of couples treated by Masters and Johnson, the cure rates for vaginismus and premature ejaculation approached 100 percent. Orgasmic dysfunction was corrected in 80 percent of women, and secondary impotence (impotence despite a history of previous coital success) resolved in 70 percent of men. Primary impotence (chronic and complete inability to maintain an erection sufficient for coitus) was cured only 60 percent of the time. Other therapists report very similar statistics.

122. The answer is C. *(Sciarra, ed 51, vol 1, chap 26, pp 1–5.)* The risk for developing breast cancer is increased by a factor of 6 by the diagnosis of atypical lobular hyperplasia. Either nulliparity or atypical ductal hyperplasia increases the risk of developing breast cancer by a factor of 3, while early menarche increases it by a factor of 1.3. There is no increase for diagnosis of sclerosing adenosis.

123. The answer is C. *(Sciarra, ed 51, vol 1, chap 26, pp 1–5.)* Approximately 80 percent of malignant breast tumors are infiltrating duct carcinomas. A bloody nipple discharge is most often due to an intraductal papilloma. Carcinoma is detected in about 18 percent of these cases, although individual studies range as high as 50 percent. Breast cysts do not increase the risk for development of breast cancer. Ninety-eight percent of breast masses are found initially by the patient, and 80 percent of breast cancers have a lump as their first symptom.

124. The answer is A. *(Speroff, ed 3. pp 370–374.)* In North America, any pubertal changes before the age of 8 years in girls and 9 years in boys are regarded as precocious. Although the most common type of precocious puberty in girls is idiopathic, it is essential to ensure close long-term follow-up of these patients to ascertain that there is not serious underlying pathology, such as tumors of the central nervous system or ovary. Only 1 to 2 percent of patients with precocious puberty have an estrogen-producing ovarian tumor as the causative factor. Albright syndrome (polyostotic fibrous dysplasia) is also relatively rare and consists of fibrous dysplasia and cystic degeneration of the long bones, sexual precocity, and café au lait spots on the skin. Hypothyroidism is a cause of precocious puberty in some children, making thyroid function tests mandatory in these cases. Central nervous system tumors as a cause of precocious puberty occur more commonly in boys than in girls.

125. The answer is E. *(Sciarra, ed 51, vol 6, chap 90, p 2.)* Risks for adverse psychological responses to gynecologic surgery include the first four answers as well as less than 12 years of formal education. The presurgical period is the most important time to sort out these factors and take necessary steps. An ideal treatment team to deal with these problems would include the gynecologist, a psychiatrist, and a nurse.

126. The answer is E. *(Speroff, ed 3. pp 114–115.)* The symptoms described in the questions are common symptoms of menopause. They all result primarily from estrogen withdrawal, and most can be reversed by estrogen therapy. "Climacteric" is actually a better word for this complex of symptoms, because the menopause is technically the instant at which menses cease.

127. The answer is E. *(Sciarra, ed 51, vol 6, chap 98, pp 2–4.)* Studies on adult sexual behavior have shown that it is the result of interactions of biological, psychological, developmental, and sociologic factors. Studies on lesbian women have been nondiagnostic in terms of finding either altered hormonal states or altered personality traits from other women. In separate surveys, 49 percent of lesbians stated "yes" they did consider having children, and the same number stated that they told their physicians of their lesbianism. Of those lesbians who did not inform their doctors of this fact, most stated that they did not because of fear of jeopardizing their medical care.

128. The answer is A. *(Kase, p 246.)* The first sign of puberty is usually the accelerated growth spurt followed by breast budding. Usually pubic hair will follow breast buds by a couple of months. Menarche is the culmination of puberty.

129. The answer is E (all). *(Kase, p 929.)* It is extremely difficult to establish if a patient-physician relationship has been created at all. There must be a contract established before responsibility for care can be imposed on the physician. It is considered appropriate for the contract to allow the patient the opportunity to accept or reject treatment proposals.

130. The answer is E (all). *(Speroff, ed 3. p 382.)* Short stature can be associated with adrenal hyperplasia, Cushing's disease, and exogenous cortisone therapy. These factors cause short stature by increasing cortisol levels and, as a result, stimulating epiphyseal closure. Individuals who have Turner syndrome also are characterized by short stature caused by a lack of estrogen production. Hypothyroidism and hypopituitarism can cause short stature in affected girls.

131. The answer is E (all). *(Speroff, ed 3. pp 116–123.)* There is good evidence that estrogen reduces anxiety, depression, and other emotional reactions that can accompany menopause. Estrogens also are helpful in retarding osteoporosis, although their use cannot replace the calcium that already has been lost. The clearest response to estrogen therapy is by the autonomic nervous system; relief from vasomotor reactions, such as hot flashes, by the use of estrogens is significant. A variety of other disturbing symptoms related to epithelial atrophy, such as dyspareunia and urinary urgency, may also be reversed with estrogen therapy.

132. The answer is E (all). *(Kase, p 247.)* Significant emotional concerns develop when puberty is delayed. By definition, if breast development has not begun by age 13, delayed puberty should be suspected. Menarche usually follows about 1 to 2 years after the beginning of breast development, and if menarche is delayed beyond age 16 delayed puberty should be investigated. Appropriate laboratory tests should be ordered. An FSH greater than 40 mIU/ml suggests hypergonadotropic hypergonadism as a cause of delayed maturation.

133. The answer is E (all). *(Masters, 1970, pp 227–237.)* Many factors can contribute to the development of primary orgasmic dysfunction in women. By definition, these women will not have been able to achieve orgasm through any physical means at any time in their lives; reasons for their dysfunction can include the influence of orthodox religious beliefs, dissatisfaction with their partners' behavioral or social traits, past trauma (such as rape), or rigid familial sexual proscriptions. Sexual dysfunction, particularly premature ejaculation in a male partner, can reinforce a woman's orgasmic dysfunction.

134. The answer is E (all). *(Kase, p 972.)* Sexual ability depends on education, experimentation, and past experience. Sexual orgasm may occur through a variety of routes: direct stimulation of the clitoris, vaginal stimulation, dreams, or stimulation of extragenital erogenous zones. There is no physiologic difference in these orgasms.

135. The answer is B (1, 3). *(Sciarra, ed 51, vol 6, chap 84, pp 1–4.)* Postpartum depression is most commonly seen in the first 3 months following delivery. Although several etiologies dealing with hormonal changes at the time of delivery have been proposed, none has yet been proven. For most women, drug therapy should not be needed, although if psychosis develops, treatment is best given by a psychiatrist. Women with past psychiatric problems are more likely to get postpartum problems, and recurrence rates as high as 50 percent are stated.

136. The answer is C (2, 4). *(Kase, p 989.)* Psychological trauma is far greater when the victim knows the rapist. The victim is less likely to report a rape when she knows the assailant and sexual dysfunction is more difficult to resolve. A woman complaining of sexual dysfunction should be carefully but gently questioned about the use of sexual force in the past.

137. The answer is E (all). *(Kase, p 975.)* Guilt or fear are known to inhibit arousal capability. There are numerous organic reasons for dyspareunia involving the vagina, uterus, ovary, or external genitalia. High estrogen pills may alter vaginal pH, leading to vaginal dryness and painful intercourse. The IUD may cause irritability that is exacerbated by intercourse.

138. The answer is E (all). *(Kase, pp 265–266.)* Dysfunctional uterine bleeding is usually a result of anovulation. Progesterone therapy followed by withdrawal will cause a sloughing of the unstable endometrium. A short-term, large-dose, combined birth-control therapy will frequently rehabilitate the bleeding endometrium. After the withdrawal bleed, the patient can be started on a low-dose cyclic combination of birth-control pills to regulate the menstrual flow. Estrogen therapy is useful on a short-term basis when the bleeding is from inadequate estrogen stimulation of endometrium. Prostaglandin synthetase inhibitors have been shown to decrease menstrual blood loss.

139. The answer is A (1, 2, 3). *(Speroff, ed 3. p 124.)* The use of estrogen replacement therapy can be deleterious for women who have thromboembolic symptoms. Because the liver is influenced significantly by estrogens, which can affect the function of hepatic cell enzymes and production of lipids and lipoproteins, the effects of hepatic impairment can be exacerbated by estrogen therapy. The existence of estrogen-dependent tumors is a contraindication to estrogen use. The long-term disabilities of osteoporosis may be ameliorated with estrogen therapy.

140. The answer is B (1, 3). *(Sciarra, ed 51, vol 6, chap 86, pp 1–4.)* Psychological symptoms during the climacteric occur at a time when much change is taking place. Hormonal levels are dropping and the menses is stopping. However, studies show these two factors not to be related to emotional symptoms in most women. Many factors, such as hormonal, environmental, and intrapsychic, combine to cause the resulting symptoms.

141–145. The answers are: 141-A, 142-E, 143-D, 144-C, 145-B. *(Romney, ed 2. pp 49–52.)* With increasing frequency physicians are called upon to become involved in the bioethical considerations of the circumstances surrounding death. The physician should be familiar with the terms used in order to better understand the debates on the moral philosophical issues of this matter. Negative or passive euthanasia is the deliberate withholding or nonadministration of an agent without which the occurrence of death and perhaps its time of occurrence are reasonably forseeable, whether it is preventable or not. Positive or active euthanasia is described as an act in which a person, other than the person dying, administers an agent that induces an intentional "good" death. Facilitated suicide is the induction of one's own death after someone else has purposefully made available the agent of death. The dying person may then exercise choice to use or not use the means of death made easily available to her or him. Suicide is the induction of one's own death by the administration of a lethal agent not intentionally procured by someone else.

Contraception, Abortion, and Sterilization

DIRECTIONS: Each question below contains five suggested responses. Select the **one best** response to each question.

146. Which of the following statements is the best explanation for the mechanism of the action of the intrauterine device (IUD)?

(A) Hyperperistalsis of the fallopian tubes accelerates the transport of the ovum, thereby preventing fertilization
(B) The IUD causes a bacterial endometritis that interferes in implantation
(C) The IUD produces menorrhagia, and the embryo is aborted in the heavy menstrual flow
(D) A sterile inflammatory reaction of the endometrium to the IUD prevents implantation
(E) A hormonal imbalance is caused by the IUD

147. The major cause of oral-contraceptive failure that results in an unplanned pregnancy is

(A) breakthrough ovulation at midcycle
(B) a high frequency of intercourse
(C) incorrect use of oral contraceptives
(D) gastrointestinal malabsorption
(E) development of antibodies

148. A pregnancy of approximately 10 weeks gestation is confirmed in a 30-year-old woman (gravida 5, para 4) with an IUD in place. The patient expresses a strong desire for the pregnancy to be continued. On examination the strings of the IUD are protruding from the cervical os. The most appropriate course of action would be to

(A) leave the IUD in place without any other treatment
(B) leave the IUD in place and continue prophylactic antibiotics throughout pregnancy
(C) remove the IUD immediately
(D) terminate the pregnancy because of the near certain risk of infection, abortion, or both
(E) perform laparoscopy to rule out an ectopic pregnancy

149. All the following statements concerning the birth-control pill and amenorrhea are true EXCEPT

(A) the incidence of postpill amenorrhea is 0.7 to 0.8 percent
(B) 80 percent of those who stop taking the pill resume normal function within 3 months
(C) 95 to 98 percent of women ovulate within 1 year of discontinuing use of the pill
(D) postpill infertility is twice the rate of infertility in those who do not use the pill
(E) women with irregular periods are more likely to develop secondary amenorrhea whether they take the pill or not

150. Techniques for second trimester abortions include all the following EXCEPT

(A) dilatation and evacuation
(B) prostaglandin E_2 vaginal suppositories
(C) intraamniotic oxytocin
(D) intraamniotic prostaglandin $F_2\alpha$
(E) intraamniotic hypertonic saline

151. The manufacture of ethinyl estradiol was an important breakthrough in the development of oral contraceptives because the agent was discovered to be

(A) an especially effective estrogen
(B) orally active
(C) less potent and therefore better tolerated than diethylstilbestrol
(D) the endogenously active form of estrogen
(E) an estrogen with a unique action on the hypothalamus

DIRECTIONS: Each question below contains four suggested responses of which **one or more** is correct. Select

A	if	**1, 2, and 3**	are correct
B	if	**1 and 3**	are correct
C	if	**2 and 4**	are correct
D	if	**4**	is correct
E	if	**1, 2, 3, and 4**	are correct

152. Which of the following is/are effective for postcoital contraception?

(1) Diethylstilbestrol, 25 mg bid for 5 days
(2) Conjugated estrogens, 30 mg for 5 days
(3) Ethinyl estradiol, 5 mg per day for 5 days
(4) Ovral, 2 tabs, PO q2h for 1 day

153. Absolute contraindications to the use of the birth-control pill include

(1) thromboembolic disorders
(2) congenital hyperlipidemia
(3) obesity and smoking in women over 35 years of age
(4) seizure disorders

154. Contraindications to the insertion of an IUD include

(1) a history of pelvic inflammatory disease
(2) previous pregnancy with an IUD
(3) abnormal genital bleeding
(4) previous cervical conization

155. Midtrimester intentional abortion by instillation of hypertonic saline into the amniotic cavity may be

(1) regulated by state law
(2) followed by Rh sensitization
(3) followed by disseminated intravascular coagulation
(4) followed by permanent hypertension

156. In patients taking combination-type birth-control pills, altered metabolic functions may include

(1) a decrease in glucose tolerance
(2) an increase in binding globulins
(3) an increase in sodium sulfobromophthalein (Bromsulphalein) retention
(4) an increase in triglycerides

157. Actual effectiveness of a given contraceptive method is less than theoretical effectiveness because of

(1) patient motivation
(2) the method's relationship to the act of coitus
(3) the method's ease of use
(4) the method's antifertility action

62

Obstetrics and Gynecology

SUMMARY OF DIRECTIONS

A	B	C	D	E
1,2,3 only	1,3 only	2,4 only	4 only	All are correct

158. The advantages of a suction curettage termination over a conventional dilatation and curettage include that the former

(1) requires less time
(2) may be performed on an outpatient
(3) has less risk of uterine perforation
(4) may be used in pregnancies in the late second trimester

159. True statements regarding operative procedures for sterilization include which of the following?

(1) They can be performed immediately post partum
(2) They have become the most common method of contraception for white couples between 20 and 40 years of age in the United States
(3) They can be considered effective immediately in females (bilateral tubal ligation)
(4) They can be considered effective immediately in males (vasectomy)

160. Progestational agents in birth-control pills have which of the following actions?

(1) Inhibition of secretion of LH
(2) Endometrial decidualization
(3) Thickening of cervical mucus
(4) Prevention of irregular menses

161. True statements concerning the estrogen component of birth-control pills include which of the following?

(1) The effect of the estrogenic agent will always take precedence over that of the progestational agent, unless the progestational agent dose is markedly increased
(2) Thromboembolic events are directly correlated with the dose of the estrogen component
(3) The estrogenic component suppresses LH secretion
(4) The estrogenic component suppresses the FSH secretion

162. A 36-year-old woman, gravida 4, para 4, presents to your office for birth-control pills. She states that she has been on the pill for 15 years without problems. She is 5'2'' tall and weighs 165 lb, her BP is 130/80, and she smokes one pack of cigarettes per day. Recommendations for birth control should include which of the following?

(1) Continuation of the birth-control pill
(2) Tubal ligation
(3) Medroxyprogesterone acetate (Depo-Provera)
(4) IUD

DIRECTIONS: Each group of questions below consists of lettered headings followed by a set of numbered items. For each numbered item select the **one** lettered heading with which it is **most** closely associated. Each lettered heading may be used **once, more than once, or not at all.**

Questions 163–166

For each method of surgical sterilization described below, select the name of the procedure.

    (A) Irving technique

    (B) Pomeroy method

    (C) Uchida method

    (D) Fimbriectomy

    (E) None of the above

163. The distal segment of the fallopian tube is removed either vaginally or abdominally

164. A plain catgut ligature is placed around a knuckle of tube, which is then excised

165. The serosa of the tube is stripped from the muscular portion and 5 cm of tube is excised; the stump is ligated and the edges of the serosa are tied around the distal tube

166. The tube is transected in the midportion and the proximal stump is buried into the myometrium

Questions 167–171

For each description that follows, select the type of abortion with which it is most commonly associated.

    (A) Spontaneous abortion

    (B) Threatened abortion

    (C) Habitual abortion

    (D) Therapeutic abortion

    (E) Elective abortion

167. The termination of pregnancy before the time of fetal viability for the purpose of safeguarding the health of the mother

168. The termination of a pregnancy before fetal viability for reasons other than maternal health or fetal disease

169. Occurrence in 10 percent of all pregnancies

170. Associated with a chromosomal anomaly in 50 to 60 percent of cases

171. Not possible with the first pregnancy

Questions 172–178

For the following methods of contraception select the most appropriate rate of use effectiveness (failure rate or percentage of pregnancies per year of actual patient use).

    (A) 80

    (B) 40

    (C) 15 to 25

    (D) 5 to 25

    (E) 3 to 10

172. Rhythm

173. IUD

174. Diaphragm

175. Postcoital douche

176. Oral contraceptive

177. Condom and spermicidal agent

178. Condom alone

Questions 179–183

For each description that follows, select the pharmacological agent with which it is most likely to be associated.

(A) Testosterone
(B) Mestranol
(C) Norethindrone
(D) Clomiphene
(E) Medroxyprogesterone acetate

179. A progestin commonly used in oral contraceptives

180. An orally active estrogen

181. An agent that at 150 mg IM every 3 months provides highly effective contraception

182. Nonsteroidal, very weak estrogen

183. An agent that causes an increase in endogenous estrogen

Questions 184–189

For each situation listed below, select the most appropriate response.

(A) Stop pills and resume after 7 days
(B) Continue pills as usual
(C) Continue pills and use an additional form of contraception
(D) Take an additional pill
(E) Stop pills and seek a medical examination

184. Nausea during first cycle of pills

185. No menses during 7 days following 21-day cycle of correct use

186. Pill forgotten for 1 day

187. Pill forgotten for 10 continuous days

188. Light bleeding at midcycle during first month on pill

189. Hemoptysis

Contraception, Abortion, and Sterilization

Answers

146. The answer is D. *(Kase, p 1038.)* It is currently believed that alteration in the cellular and biochemical components of the endometrium occurs with the IUD and an inflammatory reaction results after insertion. Polymorphonuclear leukocytes, giant cells, plasma cells, and macrophages are seen in the endometrium after exposure to all IUDs. Biochemical changes in the endometrium include changing levels of lysosomal hydrolases, glycogen deposition, oxygen composition, total proteins, acid and alkaline phosphatases, urea phospholipids, and RNA/DNA ratios. IUDs treated with copper and progesterone exert additional effects.

147. The answer is C. *(Kase, p 1010.)* The pregnancy rate with birth-control pills, based on theoretical effectiveness, is 0.1 percent. However, the pregnancy rate in actual use is 0.7 percent. This increase is due to incorrect use of the pills. Breakthrough ovulation on combination birth-control pills is thought to be a very rare occurrence. The effectiveness of the pills is not related to sexual frequency, gastrointestinal disturbances, or the development of antibodies.

148. The answer is C. *(Kase, pp 1051–1052.)* Although there is an increased risk of spontaneous abortion, and a small risk of infection, an intrauterine pregnancy can occur and continue successfully to term with an IUD in place. However, if the patient wishes to keep the pregnancy and if the strings are visible, the IUD should be removed in an attempt to reduce the risk of infection, abortion, or both. Although the percentage of ectopic pregnancies may be increased, the majority of pregnancies occurring with an IUD are intrauterine. Therefore, in the absence of signs and symptoms suggestive of an ectopic pregnancy, laparoscopy is not indicated.

149. The answer is D. *(Speroff, ed 3. p 432.)* Though the estimated incidence of "postpill amenorrhea" is given as 0.7 to 0.8 percent, there is no evidence to support the idea that oral contraception causes amenorrhea. Eighty percent of women resume normal periods within 3 months of ceasing use of the pill, and 95 to 80 percent resume normal ovulation within a year. If there were a true relationship between the pill and amenorrhea, one would expect an increase in infertility in the pill-using population. This has not been found. Infertility rates are the same for those who have used and those who have not used the pill. Patients who have not resumed normal periods 12 months after stopping use of the pill should be evaluated as any other patient with secondary amenorrhea. Women who have irregular menstrual periods are more likely to develop secondary amenorrhea whether they take the pill or not.

150. The answer is C. *(Pritchard, ed 17. pp 478–479, 482–483.)* All the methods listed in the question are used for second trimester terminations except intraamniotic oxytocin. Induction of labor with oxytocin in the second trimester requires very large doses; however, oxytocin can be used intravenously to augment contractions once labor has been initiated.

151. The answer is B. *(Speroff, ed 3. pp 410–411.)* An ethinyl group added at the 17 position makes ethinyl estradiol a very potent, orally active estrogen. Until this discovery in 1938, no orally effective estrogen had been manufactured. The effects of ethinyl estradiol on the hypothalamus and peripheral receptors are not different from those of other estrogens. Its contraceptive properties are therefore similar to those of other estrogens. Ethinyl estradiol is up to 25 times as potent as diethylstilbestrol.

152. The answer is E (all). *(Speroff, ed 3. p 442.)* Estrogen in large doses is effective as a "morning after" contraceptive. The mechanism of action is unclear. Antiemetic agents are usually prescribed to ease the nausea frequently seen as a side effect.

153. The answer is A (1, 2, 3). *(Speroff, ed 3. p 433.)* Absolute contraindications to the use of birth-control pills include (1) thromboembolic disorders (DVT, CVA, MI, or conditions predisposing to these conditions); (2) markedly impaired liver function; (3) known or suspected carcinoma of the breast or other estrogen-dependent malignancies; (4) undiagnosed abnormal genital malignancies; (4) undiagnosed abnormal genital bleeding; (5) known or suspected bleeding; (5) known or suspected pregnancy; (6) a history of obstructive jaundice in pregnancy; (7) congenital hyperlipidemia; and (8) obesity in women who are smokers and over age 35. Relative contraindications to the use of the birth-control pill require clinical judgment and informed consent. These include (1) migraine headaches; (2) hypertension; (3) uterine leiomyomata; (4) gestational diabetes; (5) elective surgery; and (6) seizure disorders.

154. The answer is B (1, 3). *(Kase, p 1047.)* A previous pregnancy with an IUD is not a contraindication to the use of an IUD. The risk of another pregnancy with the IUD in place is not increased. Previous cervical surgery in the face of a normal Pap smear and no cervical stenosis is not a contraindication to IUD use. The FDA gives the following as contraindications to the use of an IUD: (1) pregnancy; (2) pelvic inflammatory disease—acute, chronic, or recurrent; (3) acute cervicitis; (4) postpartum endometritis or septic abortion; (5) undiagnosed genital bleeding; (6) gynecologic malignancy; (7) congenital anomalies or uterine fibroids that distort the uterine cavity; and (8) copper allergy (for IUDs that contain copper). Other conditions that might preclude IUD insertion include (1) previous ectopic pregnancy; (2) severe cervical stenosis; (3) severe dysmenorrhea; (4) menometrorrhagia; (5) coagulopathies; and (6) congenital or valvular heart disease.

155. The answer is A (1, 2, 3). *(Kase, p 1063.)* Saline abortions performed in the midtrimester may be followed by significant fetomaternal transfusion. Rh_o immunoglobulin (RhoGAM) should therefore be administered to Rh-negative patients under the same conditions as with a full-term pregnancy. Although state law may not prohibit midtrimester abortions, it may regulate their performance to protect maternal health. Although they are infrequent, many serious complications may follow a saline abortion. Among these are encephalopathy, hypernatremia, hemoglobinuria, cardiac arrest, tissue necrosis, and disseminated intravascular coagulation. Although acute cardiovascular reactions, including hypertension, do occur, they are not permanent.

156. The answer is E (all.) *(Kase, pp 1018–1020.)* Combination-type oral contraceptives are potent systemic steroids that may cause many detectable alterations in metabolic function, such as increases in binding globulins, Bromsulphalein retention, triglycerides, and total phospholipids, and a decrease in glucose tolerance. Thus, the benefits of birth-control pills must be weighed carefully against the added risks in patients with diabetes, cardiovascular disease, or liver disease.

157. The answer is A (1, 2, 3). *(Kase, p 1010.)* The theoretical effectiveness is the antifertility effectiveness of the contraceptive observed under optimal conditions, that is, when used properly and regularly. Use effectiveness, on the other hand, describes the actual effectiveness observed under realistic conditions. Use effectiveness is therefore influenced by such factors as patient compliance, cost, convenience of use, side effects, relationship to coitus, and the requirement for repeated patient motivation.

158. The answer is B (1, 3). *(Kase, p 1062.)* A suction curettage can be utilized up to 12 weeks gestation. Typically, a suction curettage takes less time, has fewer major complications (including uterine perforation), and can have a lower cost. Though both conventional dilatation and curettage and suction curettage can be performed on an outpatient, the suction curettage generally requires less analgesia and is often done under local anesthesia.

159. The answer is A (1, 2, 3.) *(Kase, pp 1067–1070.)* Sterilization has become the most commonly used method of contraception in the United States for white couples between 20 and 40 years of age. In an otherwise uncomplicated pregnancy, a tubal ligation can, if desired, be performed in the immediate postpartum period. Unless the woman has already conceived at the time of the procedure, the contraceptive effect is immediate. Vasectomy in the male, however, should not be considered effective until an examination of the ejaculate is sperm-free on two successive occasions.

160. The answer is A (1, 2, 3.) *(Speroff, ed 3. pp 414–417.)* Progestational agents in oral contraceptives work by a negative-feedback mechanism to inhibit the secretion of LH and, as a result, prevent ovulation. They also cause decidualization and atrophy of the endometrium, hence making implantation impossible. In addition, cervical mucus, which at ovulation is thin and watery, is changed by the influence of progestational agents to a tenacious compound that severely limits sperm motility. Some evidence indicates that progestational agents may change ovum and sperm migration patterns within the reproductive system. Progestins do not prevent irregular bleeding. Estrogen in birth-control pills enhances the negative feedback of the progestins and stabilizes the endometrium to prevent irregular menses.

161. The answer is C (2, 4). *(Speroff, ed 3. pp 410–411, 415, 417.)* Contraceptive steroids are utilized in pharmacologic doses, not physiologic ones. Thrombosis is the most serious side effect of the pill. This side effect is directly related to the dose of estrogen. The higher the estrogen dose, the more likely there will be thrombotic complications. The combination pill prevents ovulation by inhibiting gonadotropin secretion and exerting its principal effect on pituitary and hypothalamic centers. Progesterone suppresses LH secretion while estrogen suppresses FSH secretion. The progestational effect of the pill will always take precedence over the estrogenic effect unless the estrogen dose is dramatically increased.

162.   The answer is C (2, 4). *(Speroff, ed 3. pp 419–420, 423.)* There is a known association between birth-control pills and cardiovascular death. Increased risk is not associated with duration of use. The highest risk is primarily in women over 35 who smoke and use the pill. The overall risk is very close to minimal in healthy women under the age of 40 who do not smoke, and under the age of 35 the synergistic effect of smoking may be negligible. Only smokers 35 and older have a significantly increased risk of dying from circulatory diseases. Depo-Provera is also a poor choice as a contraceptive in this obese smoker since progestin compounds decrease high-density lipoproteins (HDL) and HDL levels are inversely related to cardiovascular risk. Tubal ligation or barrier methods of contraception are the best options open to this patient.

163–166.   The answers are: 163-D, 164-B, 165-C, 166-A. *(Kase, pp 1067–1069.)* There are many surgical methods for female sterilization. Minilaparotomy and post-partum abdominal, vaginal, and laparoscopic approaches are all effective means to prevent pregnancies. Of the abdominal routes, the Pomeroy method is the most commonly used because of its simplicity and effectiveness. Laparoscopic techniques are not normally used in the immediate postpartum period.

167–171.   The answers are: 167-D, 168-E, 169-A, 170-A, 171-C. *(Pritchard, ed 17. pp 467–477.)* Abortion is defined as a pregnancy that terminates before the fetus is sufficiently developed to survive (less than 20 weeks gestation). Many different types of abortion have been identified.

Threatened abortion, signified by vaginal bleeding in early pregnancy, occurs in about 20 percent of all pregnancies. In about 50 percent of these the bleeding is secondary to implantation bleeding. These pregnancies continue in a normal fashion. The other 50 percent of threatened abortions, 10 percent of all pregnancies, result in a spontaneous abortion. A blighted ovum is the most common cause (50 percent) for spontaneous abortion. Fifty to sixty percent of early spontaneous abortions are associated with chromosomal anomalies of the conceptus.

Occasionally the products of conception will die, yet spontaneous abortion does not ensue. This prolonged retention of a dead fetus in the first half of pregnancy is termed a missed abortion. On rare occasions this prolonged retention of dead tissue can be associated with disseminated intravascular coagulation.

Habitual abortion is generally considered to be three or more consecutive spontaneous abortions. Although there are many causes for this disorder, it is probably a chance phenomenon most of the time.

A therapeutic abortion or medical abortion is one that is performed to terminate a pregnancy prior to viability for the purpose of safeguarding the health of the mother. An elective or voluntary abortion is one that is performed prior to viability at the request of the patient for reasons other than fetal or maternal health.

172–178. The answers are: 172-B, 173-E, 174-C, 175-A, 176-D, 177-D, 178-C. *(Kase, p 1011.)* There are two methods of describing the effectiveness of contraceptive agents: the theoretical or method effectiveness rate and the actual use effectiveness rate. When comparing different methods it is important to use comparable figures.

The effectiveness of the rhythm method is influenced by the woman's ability to predict the time of ovulation from the regularity of her menses. It is also influenced by the woman's motivation to successfully abstain from intercourse during the 10 days around suspected ovulation. The menstrual and ovulatory irregularities and lapses in the woman's motivation account for a pregnancy rate of 40 with the rhythm method.

In contrast to the rhythm method, the IUD requires little or no action on the part of the woman. For this reason the device's actual use effectiveness approaches its maximal theoretical effectiveness with a pregnancy rate of 3 to 10. Unrecognized expulsion or misplaced insertion of the IUD are responsible for most failures.

The vaginal diaphragm and the condom are barrier contraceptives in that for each act of sexual intercourse they pose a barrier between the sperm ejaculate and the endocervical canal. In theory, both can be very effective. However, both require recurrent motivation for application with each act of intercourse. Lapses in motivation are not uncommon, and there is a pregnancy rate of 15 to 25 for each of these two methods. The condom used with a spermicidal agent is very effective, more so than either used alone.

The pregnancy rate with postcoital douching is almost the same as that for unprotected intercourse (80). This lack of effectiveness is readily explained by the extremely rapid progression of motile sperm into the endocervical canal, coupled with the failure of a vaginal douche to reach this area.

Combined oral contraceptive birth-control pills are clearly the most effective reversible contraceptive currently available. With correct use many studies report a contraceptive effectiveness that approaches 100 percent (pregnancy rate less than 0.1). This extreme effectiveness is best explained by the pill's multiplicity of actions, i.e., suppression of ovulation, hostility of cervical mucus to sperm penetration, and hostility of atrophic endometrium to the implantation of a conceptus. Failure to take the pills with punctilious regularity is responsible for most failures.

179–183. The answers are: 179-C, 180-B, 181-E, 182-D, 183-D. *(Speroff, ed 3, pp 410–415, 439–440, 524–525.)* Ethinyl estradiol and mestranol are the two active synthetic estrogens used in birth-control pills (mestranol is employed more commonly than ethinyl estradiol). An ethinyl group at the 17 position makes these estrogens orally active.

By removing the 19 carbon from testosterone, a nontestosterone, orally active progestational agent (a 19-nortestosterone) is obtained. Norethindrone is the most commonly used progestational agent of this type in birth-control pills.

The progestational agent medroxyprogesterone acetate (Depo-Provera), along with chlormadinone, has been noted to produce benign breast tumors in beagle puppies; when estrogens were administered at the same time, however, this effect could not be reproduced. Depo-Provera is a useful alternative to the birth-control pill, especially in those women for whom estrogen is contraindicated; 150 mg IM every 3 months virtually assures 100 percent contraception. However, this method is not FDA approved.

Clomiphene is a nonsteroidal, very weak estrogenic agent. By inhibiting hypothalamic regulation of estrogen production and thus causing estrogen levels to increase, clomiphene can promote ovulation in certain groups of anovulatory women.

184–189. The answers are: 184-B, 185-B, 186-D, 187-C, 188-B, 189-E. *(Speroff, ed 3. pp 417–418, 431, 435–436.)* Common side effects of birth-control pills include nausea, breakthrough bleeding, bloating, and leg cramps. If these side effects are experienced in the first two or three cycles of pills, when they are most common, the pills may be safely continued, as these effects usually remit spontaneously.

On occasion, following correct use of a full cycle of pills, withdrawal bleeding may fail to occur (silent menses). Pregnancy is a very unlikely explanation for this event; therefore, pills should be resumed as usual (after 7 days) just as if bleeding had occurred. However, if a second consecutive period has been missed, pregnancy should be more seriously considered and ruled out by a pregnancy test, medical examination, or both.

Women occasionally forget to take pills; however, when only a single pill has been omitted, it can be taken immediately in addition to the usual pill at the usual time. This single-pill omission is associated with little if any loss in effectiveness. If three or more pills are omitted, the pill should be resumed as usual, but an additional contraceptive method (e.g., condoms) should be used through one full cycle.

Although most side effects caused by birth-control pills can be considered minor, serious side effects do sometimes occur. A painful swollen calf may signal thrombophlebitis. Hemoptysis may signal pulmonary embolism. Either of these circumstances should be considered a medical emergency, and immediate medical attention should be sought.

NORMAL PREGNANCY

The Fetus, Placenta, and Newborn

DIRECTIONS: Each question below contains five suggested responses. Select the **one best** response to each question.

190. Congenital heart malformations occur with exposure to teratogenic agents at what postmenstrual age?

(A) 2 to 3 weeks
(B) 4 to 5 weeks
(C) 6 to 8 weeks
(D) 9 to 12 weeks
(E) None of the above

191. A placenta that has a chorionic plate smaller than the basal plate is

(A) a membranaceous placenta
(B) a succenturiate placenta
(C) a circumvallate placenta
(D) a fenestrated placenta
(E) none of the above

192. The pH of a fetal scalp sample is abnormal if it is less than

(A) 7.25
(B) 7.30
(C) 7.35
(D) 7.40
(E) 7.45

193. A syndrome of multiple congenital anomalies, including microcephaly, cardiac anomalies, and growth retardation, has been described in children of women who are heavy users of

(A) amphetamines
(B) barbiturates
(C) heroin
(D) methadone
(E) ethyl alcohol

194. The finding of a single umbilical artery on examination of the umbilical cord after delivery is

(A) insignificant
(B) equal in incidence in blacks and whites
(C) an indicator of considerably increased incidence of major malformation of the fetus
(D) equally common in newborn of diabetic and nondiabetic mothers
(E) present in 5 percent of all births

195. Which of the following statements about twinning is true?

(A) The frequencies of monozygosity and dizygosity are the same
(B) Division after formation of the embryonic disc results in conjoined twins
(C) The incidence of monozygotic twinning varies with race
(D) A dichorionic twin pregnancy always denotes dizygosity
(E) Twinning confers no appreciable increase in maternal morbidity and mortality over singleton pregnancies

196. A 24-year-old primigravida presents to the obstetrics clinic at 42 weeks since the last menstrual period. The prenatal course has been benign since the first visit at 20 weeks. The blood pressure is 120/70, voided urine shows trace protein, and a vaginal examination reveals a cervix at 1 cm dilatation, 25 percent effaced, with the vertex at a −1 station. Which of the following is the most appropriate next step in the management of this patient?

(A) Ultrasound for gestational age
(B) Ultrasound for determination of amniotic fluid volume
(C) Admission to the antenatal unit for daily 24-hour urinary estriol determinations
(D) Immediate induction of labor with oxytocin
(E) Performance of nonstress test and, if reactive, follow-up with weekly vaginal examinations and induction of labor when the cervix becomes favorable

197. All the following statements about progesterone production in pregnancy are true EXCEPT

(A) progesterone production during the first 10 weeks of gestation is largely due to the corpus luteum
(B) Progesterone production after the first 12 weeks of gestation is largely due to the placenta
(C) a major substrate for placental progesterone production is maternal cholesterol
(D) progesterone levels fall rapidly with fetal demise
(E) progesterone serves as the principal substrate for fetal steroid synthesis

198. Which of the following statements concerning neural tube defects is true?

(A) The overall incidence in the United States is 2 to 3 percent
(B) Elevated maternal serum alpha-fetoprotein level is always an indicator of fetal disease
(C) Increased amniotic fluid alpha-fetoprotein levels are well correlated with severity of the lesion present
(D) Amniocentesis and detailed ultrasound evaluation of the fetus can accurately diagnose 95 to 99 percent of all cases of neural tube defects
(E) None of the above

DIRECTIONS: Each question below contains four suggested responses of which **one or more** is correct. Select

A	if	**1, 2, and 3**	are correct
B	if	**1 and 3**	are correct
C	if	**2 and 4**	are correct
D	if	**4**	is correct
E	if	**1, 2, 3, and 4**	are correct

199. A woman at 16 weeks gestation presents for a routine examination, and an ulcerative 0.5-cm lesion is observed lateral to her right labium. She reports that she has had similar irritations there for 3 years. As appropriate management steps you should

(1) verify diagnosis by culture of the lesion
(2) recommend delivery by cesarean section if lesion has healed and membranes rupture 8 hours before arrival at hospital
(3) recommend delivery by cesarean section if cervical lesions or positive cervical cultures are noted in last 4 weeks of gestation and membranes are intact
(4) recommend abortion if culture is positive because of high frequency of transplacental congenital infection in early pregnancy

200. True statements about monozygotic twinning include which of the following?

(1) It tends to run in families
(2) It frequently is associated with pregnancies induced by clomiphene citrate
(3) It is more common that dizygotic twinning
(4) It occurs in approximately 1 pregnancy in 250

201. Substances that are normally found in higher concentrations in the maternal blood than in fetal or umbilical cord blood include

(1) immunoglobulin G (IgG)
(2) immunoglobulin M (IgM)
(3) gamma chains of hemoglobin
(4) fibrinogen

202. Information about which of the following can be obtained by ultrasonography in the third trimester?

(1) Anencephaly and major neural tube defects
(2) Fetal death
(3) Polyhydramnios
(4) Most accurate dating of gestational age

203. True statements about the lecithin-to-sphingomyelin ratio include which of the following?

(1) It can reflect total muscle mass of the fetus
(2) It rises later than normal if toxemia of pregnancy has developed
(3) It rises earlier than normal if erythroblastosis fetalis has developed
(4) It can reflect fetal surfactant production

204. In humans congenital anomalies have been associated with all the following anticonvulsants EXCEPT

(1) diphenylhydantoin
(2) valproic acid
(3) trimethadione
(4) carbamazepine

205. A full-term infant is found to have a heart rate less than 100 beats per minute at 1 minute after birth. The infant does not cry and has central cyanosis, slow and irregular respiration, and some flexion of the extremities. The obstetrician should

(1) start immediate resuscitation
(2) give the infant a 1-minute Apgar score of 3
(3) call for pediatric consultation
(4) assume that adequate ventilation will correct the respiratory depression

206. Acute obstruction of the umbilical circulation has been found experimentally to provoke which of the following responses?

(1) A rapid fall in fetal central venous pressure
(2) An almost immediate fall in fetal heart rate
(3) A rapidly mediated humoral effect on the fetal heart
(4) A rapidly mediated response by the fetal heart that can be affected by cutting the vagi

207. Severe fetal or neonatal infection can result from maternal infection near term by which of the following viruses?

(1) Group B coxsackievirus
(2) Rubella virus
(3) Chickenpox virus
(4) Herpesvirus hominis, type 2

208. Maternal diabetes mellitus is associated with which of the following symptoms in the fetus or neonate?

(1) Macrosomia in the fetus
(2) Delayed pulmonic maturity in the fetus
(3) Hypoglycemia in the newborn
(4) Hypocalcemia in the newborn

209. True statements about the twin-twin transfusion syndrome include which of the following?

(1) The donor twin develops hydramnios more often than does the recipient twin
(2) Gross differences may be observed between donor and recipient placentas
(3) The donor twin usually suffers from a hemolytic anemia
(4) The recipient twin can develop widespread thromboses

SUMMARY OF DIRECTIONS

A	B	C	D	E
1,2,3 only	1,3 only	2,4 only	4 only	All are correct

210. True statements about twins include that

(1) perinatal mortality for twin fetuses is higher than that for singletons
(2) an increased risk of death for twins persists only for 1 month post partum
(3) the perinatal mortality for monozygous twins is higher than that for dizygous twins
(4) intrauterine death from cord accidents is a rare cause of death in monoamniotic twins

211. An infant is likely to be compromised as a result of vaginal delivery that is accompanied by which of the following conditions?

(1) Prolapse of the umbilical cord
(2) Shoulder presentation
(3) Persistent brow presentation
(4) Persistent occiput posterior position

212. True statements describing toxoplasmosis in a pregnant woman include which of the following?

(1) It can be acquired by eating infected raw meat
(2) It occurs in 1 in every 2000 to 2500 pregnancies
(3) Infection in early pregnancy may lead to abortion
(4) Transplacental infection of the fetus is highly unlikely

213. The human placenta produces which of the following hormones?

(1) Gonadotropin
(2) Somatomammotropin
(3) Progesterone
(4) Hydrocortisone

214. Situations that increase the risk of morbidity or mortality for the fetus of a diabetic mother include

(1) maternal ketoacidosis
(2) maternal ketonuria in the absence of diabetic ketoacidosis
(3) maternal hyperglycemia
(4) maternal hypoglycemia

215. Chorioangiomas can be described by which of the following statements?

(1) They affect more than 5 percent of placentas
(2) They often are associated with anomalous cord insertions
(3) They often are associated with cords containing only two vessels
(4) They are the most common tumors of the placenta

216. Substances that cross the placenta poorly or not at all include

(1) thyroxine
(2) long-acting thyroid stimulator
(3) thyroid-stimulating hormone
(4) propylthiouracil

DIRECTIONS: The group of questions below consists of lettered headings followed by a set of numbered items. For each numbered item select the **one** lettered heading with which it is **most** closely associated. Each lettered heading may be used **once, more than once, or not at all.**

Questions 217–220

For each of the following substances, choose the mechanism of transplacental transport most likely to be employed.

(A) Simple diffusion
(B) Facilitated diffusion
(C) Active transport
(D) Pinocytosis
(E) None of the above

217. Carbon dioxide

218. Iron

219. Oxygen

220. Glucose

The Fetus, Placenta, and Newborn

Answers

190. The answer is C. *(Danforth, ed 4. pp 316–318.)* Streeter hypothesized that each organ system has a definite time for appearance and differentiation. Consequently, when an insult occurs, it cannot affect or alter a structure that has differentiated earlier or one that does not develop until after the insult is completed. Major heart and circulatory structures are found from 6 to 8 weeks postmenstrual age.

191. The answer is C. *(Pritchard, ed 17. pp 441–442.)* Abnormalities of placentation in which the chorionic plate is smaller than the basal plate include circumvallate and circummarginate placentas, and they are known as extrachorial placentas. Succenturiate placentas have accessory lobes in the membrane away from the main body of the placenta, and they are connected by large vessels to the main body. A membranaceous placenta has functioning villi covering all the fetal membranes, and a fenestrated placenta is one in which the central portion of the placenta is missing.

192. The answer is A. *(Pritchard, ed 17. p 288.)* A fetal scalp pH of 7.20 to 7.24 is borderline abnormal and should be repeated within 30 minutes unless delivery intervenes. If the pH is less than 7.20, immediate collection of a confirmatory sample is necessary with movement toward prompt delivery if the low pH is continued; otherwise, labor may continue with repeat sampling periodically.

193. The answer is E. *(Burrow, ed 2. pp 450–451.)* Chronic alcohol abuse, which can cause liver disease, folate deficiency, and many other disorders in a pregnant woman, also can lead to the development of congenital abnormalities in the child. The chief abnormalities associated with the fetal alcohol syndrome are microcephaly, growth retardation, and cardiac anomalies. Chronic abuse of alcohol also may be associated with an increased incidence of mental retardation in the children of affected women.

194. The answer is C. *(Pritchard, ed 17. p 459.)* The absence of one umbilical artery occurs in 0.7 to 0.8 percent of all umbilical cords of singletons, in 2.5 percent of all abortuses, and in approximately 5 percent of at least one twin. The incidence of a single artery is significantly increased in newborns of diabetic mothers, and it occurs in white infants twice as often as in newborns of black women. The incidence of major fetal malformations when only one artery is identified has been reported as high as 18 percent, and there is an increased incidence of overall fetal mortality.

195. The answer is B. *(Pritchard, ed 17. pp 503–506.)* The incidence of mono-zygotic twinning is constant at a rate of one set per 250 births around the world. It is unaffected by race, heredity, age, parity, or infertility agents. Examination of the amnion and chorion can be used to determine monozygosity only if one chorion is identified. Two identifiable chorions can occur in monozygotic or dizygotic twin-ning. The time of the division of a fertilized zygote to form monozygotic twins determines the placental and membranous anatomy. Late division after formation of the embryonic disc will result in conjoined twins.

196. The answer is B. *(Pritchard, ed 17. pp 761–764.)* The management of post-term pregnancy is always controversial, and it is often complicated by questionable dates and a cervix that is unfavorable for induction. Immediate induction of an unfavorable cervix is not always successful, and it may expose the patient to in-creased morbidity and mortality from an unnecessary cesarean section. Reliance on dating by the last menstrual period alone always leaves a question of true postma-turity of the fetus and can pose a risk if labor is induced in what is actually a premature infant. Ultrasound for amniotic fluid volume is appropriate in this case because it indicates fetal well-being near term, especially when combined with an-tenatal fetal heart rate testing. Urinary estriol levels have not proven to be an accurate indicator of fetal distress in postdate management. Any protocol that involves fetal heart rate testing must be performed on a regular basis, and it should involve some type of contraction stress testing for optimal results.

197. The answer is D. *(Speroff, ed 3. p 272.)* The corpus luteum constitutes the major source of progesterone production during the first 10 weeks of pregnancy. The placenta represents the major source of progesterone production after the first 12 weeks. As the placenta is unable to synthesize cholesterol from acetate, the major substrate for placental progesterone production comes from maternal cholesterol. Fetal synthesis of progesterone contributes little to the maternal levels; therefore, progesterone levels will remain high, even after fetal demise. The most important role of progesterone in the fetus is as a substrate for fetal adrenal gland production of gluco- and mineralocorticoids.

198. The answer is D. *(Burrow, ed 2. pp 121–122.)* The overall incidence of neural tube defects in the United States is 1 to 2 per 1000 live births. However, a mother with a previous child with a neural tube defect has a recurrent risk ranging from 1.7 to 6 percent. Maternal serum alpha-fetoprotein levels vary with gestational age. When elevated above the level appropriate for gestational age, they may be associated with numerous other problems, including multiple gestation, threatened abortion, intrauterine demise, Rh disease, ectopic pregnancy, maternal or neonatal hepatitis, maternal hepatoma, gastrointestinal cancer, tumor metastatic to the liver, maternal herpes infection, fetal congenital cirrhosis, fetal tyrosinosis, preeclampsia, fetal growth retardation, and other major malformations, such as omphalocele, nephrosis, or esophageal atresia. Amniotic fluid alpha-fetoprotein would be elevated in 90 percent of all infants with neural tube defects, but the concentration does not correlate with the severity of the disease. A fetus with a closed defect may not show an increased alpha-fetoprotein level in the amniotic fluid, and elevated levels may return to normal at 24 weeks gestational age, even if a fetus does have an open neural tube defect. However, amniocentesis combined with a detailed ultrasound evaluation of the fetal spine should accurately diagnose 95 to 99 percent of all cases.

199. The answer is B (1, 3). *(Burrow, ed 2. pp 356–357.)* A suspicious genital lesion in pregnancy must be cultured for herpesvirus; if culture is positive, examination for lesions and cervical cultures are mandatory in the last month of pregnancy. Transplacental or ascending infection of the fetus with intact membranes is rare. Delivery by cesarean section is recommended for active lesions or positive culture within 2 to 4 weeks of delivery if membranes have been ruptured for less than 4 hours. Longer rupture probably exposes the fetus prior to delivery and abdominal delivery will not ensure safety. Conversely, with negative culture and absence of lesions, vaginal delivery can be undertaken with reasonable safety.

200. The answer is D (4). *(Pritchard, ed 17. pp 503–504.)* Monozygotic twins are formed from the splitting of a single fertilized ovum and occur in approximately 1 birth in 250. Dizygotic twins, which are more common, result from multiple ovulations during the same menstrual cycle. The incidence of monozygotic twinning seems to be relatively constant despite differences in race, heredity, age, and hormonal therapy. Dizygotic twinning, on the other hand, is influenced by all these factors; it occurs more commonly in blacks than in whites, seems to run (by the maternal-hereditary line) in families, and is more common with increasing age and parity. The use of clomiphene for ovulation induction is associated with multiple ovulation and an approximately 7 percent incidence of multiple gestation (as opposed to approximately 1.0 to 1.4 percent in the normal population). The use of gonadotropins to stimulate ovulation is associated with an even higher incidence of multiple gestations, with some series reporting as high as 40 percent.

201. The answer is C (2, 4). *(Pritchard, ed 17. pp 151–153.)* Immunoglobulin G (IgG) easily crosses the placenta and thus is found in approximately equal amounts in maternal and fetal blood. Immunoglobulin M (IgM), on the other hand, is a large molecule and does not cross the placenta. Thus maternal levels of IgM are higher than fetal levels, unless an intrauterine infection causes the fetus to manufacture IgM. The gamma chains in hemoglobin (Hb) are what distinguish fetal hemoglobin from adult hemoglobin. Fetal hemoglobin (Hb F) contains two alpha and two gamma chains. Hb A, found in most adults, contains two alpha and two beta chains. One would therefore expect to find more gamma chains in the fetal blood than in maternal blood. Finally, cord-blood fibrinogen levels are normally quite low; maternal fibrinogen levels, on the other hand, are about 50 percent higher than levels in nonpregnant women.

202. The answer is A (1, 2, 3). *(Jeanty, pp 45, 55–67, 99–105.)* Determination of fetal age using biparietal diameter is most accurate before the 26th week when the rate of growth is faster and the variation among fetuses of the same age is less. Fetal death can be diagnosed by lack of limb or heart motion, irregularity of skull outline, or excessive flexion in posture. Polyhydramnios is characterized by increased uterine volume with extensive echo-free areas. Many neural tube defects and anencephaly can be diagnosed by abnormalities in the skull and spine on ultrasound.

203. The answer is D (4). *(Burrow, ed 2. pp 97–98.)* The lecithin-to-sphingomyelin (L/S) ratio, measured from amniotic-fluid samples, is a barometer of pulmonic maturity. If the L/S ratio is above whatever value denotes maturity in a particular laboratory, respiratory distress syndrome will probably not be present in the newborn. Lecithin seems to be involved in surfactant activity, and its secretion from the lungs into the amniotic fluid yields information about surfactant production in the fetal lungs. Amniotic-fluid creatinine values have been used to document fetal maturity; but because they also can reflect the muscle mass of a fetus, they are not as valid as the L/S ratio. The L/S ratio may reach maturity levels earlier in stressful situations, as in toxemia of pregnancy. Delay in pulmonic maturation occurs in association with mild diabetes but not with erythroblastosis fetalis.

204. The answer is D (4). *(Burrow, ed 2. pp 430–439.)* Fetal hydantoin syndrome is characterized by craniofacial anomalies, deficient growth, mental retardation, and limb defects. Valproic acid has been associated with increased risks of neural tube defects. Trimethadione-affected infants have developmental delay, low-set ears, palate anomalies, irregular teeth, V-shaped eyebrows, and speech disturbances. Although carbamazepine has been associated with hematological problems in patients, no reports of teratogenicity have been published. When possible, a seizure-free woman should be withdrawn from medication before pregnancy, but if she is actively epileptic, continued therapy is advised because of the danger of prolonged seizures.

205. The answer is A (1, 2, 3). *(Pritchard, ed 17. pp 381–383.)* The assessment tool for infants known as the Apgar score is based on the infant's condition 1 minute and 5 minutes after birth. Heart rate, respiratory effort, muscle tone, reflex irritability, and body color are assessed. The maximum score is 10 (2 points per category), and the lowest score is 0. A perfect score indicates heart rate greater than 100 beats per minute, good respiratory effort, active motion, vigorous crying, and pink body color. Responses that are present but not optimal earn a score of 1 per category, while an absence of response gives no score. Apgar scores of 4 to 7 at 1 minute indicate mild respiratory depression; infants who score under 4 are severely depressed. Thus, a low 1-minute Apgar score indicates the need for immediate resuscitation, and a low 5-minute Apgar score indicates increased risk of morbidity and mortality. The infant presented in the question is severely depressed, and the physician should assume nothing regarding resuscitation.

206. The answer is C (2, 4). *(Aladjem, ed 2. pp 56–62.)* Fetal heart rate has been shown to drop almost immediately when the umbilical circulation has been obstructed in experimental situations. This response is a reflex action that is caused by the sudden rise in central venous pressure and that disappears if the vagi are severed. A more prolonged obstruction of the umbilical circulation can cause a delayed fall in the fetal heart rate secondary to progressive asphyxia.

207. The answer is E (all). *(Burrow, ed 2. pp 333–346.)* A mild group B coxsackievirus infection of the mother during the antepartum period may give rise to a virulent infection in the newborn, sometimes resulting in a fatal encephalomyocarditis. A maternal rubella infection may cause neonatal hepatosplenomegaly, petechial rash, and jaundice; in addition, viral shedding may last for months or years. Herpes zoster, the causative agent of varicella (chickenpox), is an especially dangerous organism for the newborn. Varicella is rare in pregnancy, but if it occurs shortly before delivery, the viremia may spread to the fetus before protective maternal antibodies have had a chance to form. Congenital varicella can be fatal to the newborn; the increasing availability of zoster immunoglobulin, however, may allow clinicians to attack the infection before significant fetal viremia has developed. Herpesvirus can be acquired by the fetus as it passes down the genital tract and can cause a severe, often fatal herpes infection in the newborn.

208. The answer is E (all). *(Burrow, ed 2. pp 48–50.)* Maternal diabetes, especially of the milder classes, is associated with macrosomia in the fetus. Glucose crosses the placenta freely by facilitated diffusion, but insulin does not. The fetus, in response to the chronic glucose load, secretes increased quantities of insulin. Insulin acts as a growth hormone in the fetus, and the fetus becomes macrosomic. At delivery, the fetus is removed from the relatively glucose-rich maternal environment but continues to secrete increased amounts of insulin. Thus, the fetus may become hypoglycemic in the early hours of life unless early feedings, sometimes even intravenous glucose, are begun. Hypocalcemia may occur in as many as one fourth of infants of diabetic mothers, possibly as a result of fetal parathyroid suppression stemming from maternal hypercalcemia. Lastly, fetal lung maturity, as measured by the lecithin-to-sphingomyelin ratio, may be delayed, especially in the infants of mothers who have mild diabetes.

209. The answer is C (2, 4). *(Benirschke, NY State J Med 61:4499, 1961.)* In the twin-twin transfusion syndrome, the donor twin is always anemic, owing not to a hemolytic process but to the direct transfer of blood to the recipient twin. The recipient may suffer thromboses secondary to hypertransfusion and subsequent hemoconcentration. Although the donor placenta is usually pale and somewhat atrophied, that of the recipient is congested and enlarged. Hydramnios can develop in either twin but, because of circulatory overload, is more frequent in the recipient. Hydramnios when it occurs in the donor is due to congestive heart failure caused by severe anemia.

210. The answer is B (1, 3). *(Pritchard, ed 17. pp 513–514.)* The mortality for twins remains higher than for singletons throughout the first year and only approaches that of singletons in the second year. Intertwining of umbilical cords is a common cause of death in monoamniotic twins. However, even for monozygotic twins, most are *not* monoamniotic.

211. The answer is A (1, 2, 3). *(Pritchard, ed 17. pp 658–668.)* Shoulder presentation, either as a transverse or an oblique lie, presents significant problems when vaginal delivery of an affected infant is attempted because the shoulder is arrested by the margins of the pelvic inlet. Similarly, persistent brow presentation compromises the infant because the resultant extensive molding deforms the head. The presence of a prolapsed umbilical cord is also associated with significant compromise of infants delivered vaginally since the cord becomes compressed between the presenting part and the margin of the pelvic inlet. Persistent occiput posterior position does not significantly compromise an infant during the course of a normal vaginal delivery.

212. The answer is B (1, 3). *(Pritchard, ed 17. p 787.)* Toxoplasmosis, a protozoal infection caused by *Toxoplasma gondii,* can result from ingestion of raw or under-cooked meat infected by the organism or from contact with infected cat feces. Its incidence in pregnant women is estimated to be 1 in every 150 to 700 pregnancies. Infection early in pregnancy may cause abortion; later in pregnancy, however, the fetus may become infected. A small number of infected infants develop involvement of the central nervous system or the eye; most infants who have the disease, however, escape serious clinical problems.

213. The answer is A (1, 2, 3). *(Pritchard, ed 17. pp 119–123, 133–135.)* The polypeptide hormones human chorionic gonadotropin (HCG) and human chorionic somatomammotropin (HCS) are produced by the syncytiotrophoblast of the human placenta. Because these hormones reflect placental rather than fetal integrity, the presence of HCG in the urine or blood may persist after fetal death (in the case of missed abortion) and even after spontaneous or therapeutic abortion. HCG is im-munologically quite similar to pituitary luteinizing hormone (LH), the difference being in the amino acid sequence of the beta subunit. This fact must be considered when interpreting results of pregnancy tests based on HCG bioassay, results that are not always positive until 42 days gestation. The specific immunoassay for the beta subunit of HCG, on the other hand, may be positive even before a menstrual period is missed. Progesterone is made in large amounts by the placenta. There is no good evidence to support a placental role in the production of adrenocorticosteroids.

214. The answer is A (1, 2, 3). *(Burrow, ed 2. p 50.)* Sophisticated management of high-risk diabetic individuals has reduced the incidence of diabetic ketoacidosis. When it occurs in pregnant women, however, it is associated with an extremely high fetal mortality. In addition, ketonuria in the absence of acidosis (i.e., starvation ketosis) has been correlated with decreased intelligence quotients in the offspring. Perinatal mortality has been correlated with hyperglycemia even in the absence of ketoacidosis, and this finding is the cornerstone of current recommendations urging strict control of diabetes during pregnancy. A correlation between maternal hypo-glycemia and fetal morbidity or mortality has not been shown; in fact, rather severe episodes of hypoglycemia have been reported to have no effect on the outcome of pregnancy.

215. The answer is D (4). *(Aladjem, ed 2. p 284.)* Chorioangiomas are the most common placental tumor, occurring in approximately 1 percent of placentas. Despite attempts to correlate the presence of this tumor with hydramnios and fetal anomalies, no significant effect on fetal morbidity and mortality has been demonstrated, unless the size of the tumor is very great.

216. The answer is B (1, 3). *(Burrow, ed 2. pp 195, 204.)* Thyroxine crosses the placenta poorly, if at all. For this reason, a hyperthyroid mother does not transmit her hyperthyroidism to the fetus, and giving thyroid hormone to a hypothyroid mother will not raise fetal thyroxine levels significantly. Thyroid-stimulating hormone (TSH) also does not cross to the fetus. On the other hand, propylthiouracil (PTU), an antithyroid drug, crosses easily and may suppress fetal thyroid function. Hyperthyroid women taking large doses of PTU therefore run the risk of having goitrous babies. Some clinicians, hoping to reverse the effect of PTU on the fetus, have given thyroxine to the mother; theoretically, however, this should not work, because the thyroid hormone should not get to the fetus. Long-acting thyroid stimulator (LATS) is present in many patients who have Graves' disease. Because LATS can cross the placenta, LATS levels should be obtained from such patients and the pediatrician should be alerted to possible neonatal thyrotoxicosis if LATS is present.

217–220. The answers are: 217-A, 218-C, 219-A, 220-B. *(Pritchard, ed 17. pp 147–149, 167–169.)* Oxygen travels from mother to fetus, and carbon dioxide from fetus to mother, by *simple diffusion* across the placenta. Carbon dioxide travels more rapidly than oxygen, probably because fetal and maternal blood have different affinities for these two substances. Iron is *actively transported* (i.e., in an energy-requiring process) from mother to fetus; as a result, the mother may become markedly iron-depleted during pregnancy, while the fetus does well. Glucose crosses to the fetus by *facilitated diffusion,* which means that its transfer across the placenta is more rapid than could be accounted for by simple diffusion alone. The fetus acts as a "glucose sink," continuously obtaining glucose at the expense of the mother. This fact may help to explain the lower-than-normal levels of maternal fasting blood glucose found during pregnancy. *Pinocytosis* describes the process by which liquid is imbibed by cells as a result of invagination of the cell membrane.

Pregnancy, Labor, Delivery, and Puerperium

DIRECTIONS: Each question below contains five suggested responses. Select the **one best** response to each question.

221. Normal values for thyroid function tests increase during pregnancy in all the following tests EXCEPT

(A) basal metabolic rate
(B) total thyroxine
(C) total triiodothyronine
(D) radioiodine uptake (percent)
(E) free thyroxine

Questions 222–224

The sketch shown below details the major landmarks of the fetal skull as it presents in the maternal pelvis. The perspective is that of the obstetrician facing the perineum.

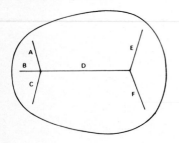

222. The position of the fetal vertex is

(A) left occiput anterior
(B) left sacrum transverse
(C) left occiput transverse
(D) right occiput transverse
(E) mentum posterior

223. The lambdoid sutures are

(A) **A** and **C**
(B) **A, C,** and **D**
(C) **B** and **D**
(D) **E** and **F**
(E) none of the above

224. The intersection of **D, E,** and **F** forms the

(A) caput succedaneum
(B) parietal prominence
(C) biparietal plane
(D) anterior fontanelle
(E) posterior fontanelle

225. The pH of amniotic fluid is

(A) 2.5 to 3.0
(B) 3.0 to 3.5
(C) 4.5 to 5.5
(D) 5.5 to 6.0
(E) 7.0 to 7.5

226. An abnormal attitude is illustrated by

(A) breech
(B) face presentation
(C) transverse position
(D) occiput posterior
(E) occiput anterior

227. Coitus in pregnancy has been shown to

(A) increase the incidence of preterm births
(B) be of lower frequency than in the nonpregnant state
(C) be more likely to result in orgasm than in the nonpregnant state
(D) increase the incidence of uterine infections
(E) result in contractions only if orgasm is reached

228. In normal pregnancy alpha-fetoprotein levels

(A) are highest in amniotic fluid
(B) decrease after the first trimester in both the fetus and amniotic fluid
(C) in maternal serum change proportionally with those in the fetus through pregnancy
(D) are produced exclusively in the fetal liver
(E) when found to be abnormally elevated, are a specific marker for neural tube defects

229. A pregnant woman is seen 18 days after she has been exposed to rubella. Her hemagglutination inhibition titer is 1:8. Her physician should

(A) administer rubella vaccine
(B) recommend an abortion
(C) repeat the titer 2 days later
(D) repeat the titer 10 to 14 days later
(E) obtain weekly titers for the next 4 weeks

230. The oxytocin challenge test is considered negative if

(A) at least three uterine contractions occur in a 10-minute interval and late deceleration of fetal heart rate is absent
(B) at least three uterine contractions occur in a 10-minute interval and late deceleration is inconsistent
(C) less than three uterine contractions occur in a 10-minute interval, regardless of whether late deceleration occurs
(D) the uterus contracts at least once every 2 minutes, regardless of whether late deceleration occurs
(E) no uterine contractions are noted

231. The smallest anteroposterior diameter of the pelvic inlet is called

(A) interspinous diameter
(B) true conjugate
(C) diagonal conjugate
(D) obstetric conjugate
(E) none of the above

232. A pregnant woman is discovered to be an asymptomatic carrier of *Neisseria gonorrhoeae*. A year ago, she was treated with penicillin for a gonococcal infection and developed a severe allergic reaction. Treatment of choice at this time would be

(A) tetracycline
(B) ampicillin
(C) spectinomycin
(D) chloramphenicol
(E) none of the above

233. The major reason that birth-control pills are contraindicated for lactating mothers is their association with

(A) fibrocystic disease of the breast
(B) carcinoma of the breast
(C) thromboembolism in the newborn
(D) subsequent onset of juvenile diabetes
(E) jaundice in the newborn

234. A 25-year-old woman, gravida 1, para 0, who has a history of infertility, comes to your office at 20 weeks gestation. Her uterus is enlarged (24 weeks). She was treated in the past with a fertility drug, the name of which she does not know. You obtain an ultrasonogram, which is shown below. The most likely diagnosis is

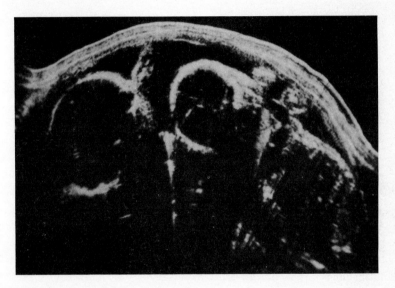

(A) hydatidiform mole
(B) placenta previa
(C) anencephalic fetus
(D) twins
(E) normal single-fetus pregnancy

235. The x-ray shown below, which
was taken in the plane of the pelvic inlet, demonstrates which of the following types of pelvic morphology?

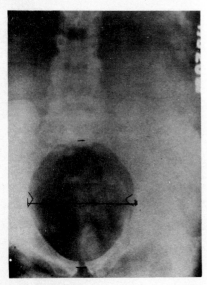

(A) Anthropoid
(B) Android
(C) Gynecoid
(D) Platypelloid
(E) Trianguloid

DIRECTIONS: Each question below contains four suggested responses of which **one or more** is correct. Select

A	if	**1, 2, and 3**	are correct
B	if	**1 and 3**	are correct
C	if	**2 and 4**	are correct
D	if	**4**	is correct
E	if	**1, 2, 3, and 4**	are correct

236. Agents that cause uterine contractions include which of the following?

(1) Ergonovine maleate (Ergotrate)
(2) Oxytocin (Pitocin)
(3) Methylergonovine maleate (Methergine)
(4) Prostaglandin E_2

237. High resting intrauterine pressures can be seen with which of the following?

(1) Placental abruption
(2) Cephalopelvic disproportion
(3) Oxytocin (Pitocin) hyperstimulation
(4) Fetal malpresentation

238. The use of aspirin in pregnancy may be associated with which of the following complications?

(1) Polyhydramnios
(2) Maternal platelet dysfunction
(3) Premature labor
(4) Neonatal jaundice

239. True statements about $Rh_0(D)$ immune globulin (RhoGAM) include which of the following?

(1) Administration is therapeutically unsuccessful in approximately 1.5 percent of cases
(2) It should never be administered during pregnancy
(3) It usually is given in a dose of 300 μg within 72 hours of delivery of an Rh-positive infant to an unsensitized Rh-negative woman
(4) It can prevent ABO (blood group) incompatibility

240. Women at risk for a suboptimal nutritional state while pregnant include those

(1) in a low socioeconomic group
(2) less than age 16
(3) underweight at the start of pregnancy
(4) having a third pregnancy within a 2-year time span

241. Appropriate measures in the treatment of women who have edema of pregnancy include

(1) salt restriction
(2) weight control
(3) diuretics
(4) bed rest

SUMMARY OF DIRECTIONS

A	B	C	D	E
1,2,3 only	1,3 only	2,4 only	4 only	All are correct

242. Which of the following circumstances should alert an obstetrician to an increased likelihood of postpartum hemorrhage?

(1) Prolonged labor
(2) Rapid labor
(3) Oxytocin stimulation of labor
(4) Twin pregnancy

243. Advantages of the McDonald cerclage over the Shirodkar procedure to treat cervical incompetence include which of the following?

(1) A higher success rate is achieved
(2) There is less scarring of the cervix
(3) Nonabsorbable suture is used
(4) It is a technically easier procedure

244. Following a cesarean birth, contraindications for a trial of labor in a subsequent pregnancy include

(1) the lack of a prior vaginal delivery
(2) the fact that the first section was for cephalopelvic disproportion (CPD)
(3) the inavailability of x-ray pelvimetry
(4) a classic c-section scar

245. True statements about the oxytocin challenge test (also called the contraction stress test) include which of the following?

(1) It determines the inducibility of the uterus
(2) Its effects are measured by internal monitors
(3) It is considered positive if the uterus contracts once every 2 minutes
(4) It can serve as a fetal stress test

246. Potential treatments for use in the initial care of late postpartum hemorrhage include

(1) methylergonovine maleate (Methergine)
(2) oxytocin injection (Pitocin)
(3) ergonovine maleate (Ergotrate)
(4) prostaglandins

247. Side effects seen with conduction anesthesia include

(1) hypotension
(2) bladder dysfunction
(3) postpartum headaches
(4) hypertension following Methergine administration

248. Electronic fetal monitoring is used to assess fetal well-being during labor. Patterns associated with fetal compromise include which of the following?

(1) Loss of beat-to-beat variability
(2) Persistent fetal tachycardia
(3) Late decelerations
(4) Variable decelerations

249. The use of which of the following antibiotics is contraindicated during pregnancy?

(1) Tetracycline
(2) Penicillin
(3) Chloramphenicol
(4) Ampicillin

DIRECTIONS: The group of questions below consists of lettered headings followed by a set of numbered items. For each numbered item select the **one** lettered heading with which it is **most** closely associated. Each lettered heading may be used **once, more than once, or not at all.**

Questions 250–254

The safety of immunization during pregnancy is a matter of concern and controversy that has prompted the American College of Obstetricians and Gynecologists to offer specific recommendations for the use of immunization therapy for pregnant women. For each disease vaccine listed below, select the recommendation with which it is most likely to be associated.

(A) Recommended if the underlying disease is serious
(B) Recommended after exposure or before travel to endemic areas
(C) Not routinely recommended but mandatory during an epidemic
(D) Contraindicated unless exposure to the disease is unavoidable
(E) Contraindicated

250. Poliomyelitis

251. Mumps

252. Influenza

253. Rubella

254. Hepatitis A

Pregnancy, Labor, Delivery, and Puerperium

Answers

221. The answer is E. *(Pritchard, ed 17. pp 202–203.)* Thyroid-binding globulin levels are increased in pregnancy. This is an effect of elevated levels of estrogen and is also seen in patients taking exogenous estrogens, such as oral contraceptives. Therefore there is an increase in total T4 and T3 along with a decrease in T3 resin uptake. Despite the increased total values of thyroid hormones, unbound or free, T4 and T3 values remain unchanged. There is a 25 percent increase in the basal metabolic rate. There is an increase in radioiodine uptake, but this test should not be performed in pregnancy because of the deleterious effects of radioactive iodine on the fetus.

222–224. The answers are: 222-C, 223-D, 224-E. *(Pritchard, ed 17. p 237.)* A good knowledge of the major landmarks of the fetal skull is essential for anyone performing deliveries. The position of the fetal vertex in the sketch accompanying the question is left occiput transverse. The lambdoid sutures (**E** and **F**) meet the sagittal suture (**D**) to form the posterior fontanelle. The occiput is just posterior to the posterior fontanelle. The posterior, or Y-shaped, fontanelle is the reference point for vertex presentations. The side of the maternal pelvis to which it is closest defines the position. The head is oriented in a transverse (or horizontal) manner, with the occiput nearest the maternal left side; thus, this is left occiput transverse. The anterior, or diamond-shaped, fontanelle, is made up of the intersection of the sagittal, frontal (**B**), and the two coronal (**A** and **C**) sutures. Extreme molding of the fetal head may make identification of these landmarks very difficult. Other clues to the position of the head include abdominal palpation of the back and small parts and, more important, palpation of an ear. If an ear can be felt and the relationship between the locations of the pinna and the auditory canal can be ascertained, the position of the vertex can be deduced.

225. The answer is E. *(Pritchard, ed 17. p 333.)* The pH of amniotic fluid is generally 7.0 to 7.5. The pH of the vagina is 4.5 to 5.5. This distinction forms the basis of the nitrazine test to diagnose rupture of the membranes.

226. The answer is B. *(Pritchard, ed 17. p 235.)* Lie of the fetus refers to the relation of the long axis of the fetus to that of the mother and is classified as longitudinal, transverse, or oblique. The fetal attitude refers to the fetal posture—either flexed or extended. A face presentation results from an extension of the fetus at the neck. Presentation refers to the portion of the baby that is foremost in the birth canal. Occiput transverse and occiput anterior are examples of positions, that is, relative relationship of the fetus to the mother.

227. The answer is E. *(Sciarra, ed 51, vol 2, chap 20, pp 4–5.)* Coitus is often cited as a cause of infection in preterm birth, although this relationship has not been proven. Both the frequency of coitus and the chance that it will result in orgasm are decreased in pregnant women. Contractions are noted when pregnant women reach orgasm.

228. The answer is B. *(Pritchard, ed 17. p 277.)* Alpha-fetoprotein is the major serum protein of the early fetus. It is produced in the yolk sac and fetal liver. Levels in the fetus and amniotic fluid increase until approximately 13 weeks and then drop off until term. Maternal levels, however, slowly increase until late pregnancy. Levels in the fetus are approximately 150 times those found in the amniotic fluid and up to 1000 times those in the maternal serum. Abnormal elevations of alpha-fetoprotein are seen in pregnancies complicated by neural tube defects, low birthweight, fetal distress, and gastrointestinal abnormalities, as well as other conditions. Elevated alpha-fetoprotein levels are a sensitive, but not specific, marker of neural tube defects.

229. The answer is D. *(Burrow, ed 2. pp 335–337.)* A titer of 1:8 obtained by a hemagglutination inhibition test may or may not indicate prior exposure to rubella virus. This titer in an exposed patient could represent a false positive result caused by the presence of nonspecific hemagglutinin inhibitors, which can be found in all human sera. On the other hand, a patient who has a titer of 1:8 18 days after exposure to rubella could be susceptible and harboring an inapparent infection that has just begun to stimulate manufacture of antibody. If a titer repeated 10 to 14 days later is the same as the first one, the patient is assumed to be immune. If, on the other hand, the repeat titer is 1:32 or greater, the initial titer most likely represented early antibody response to an inapparent infection. Rubella vaccination is contraindicated in pregnant women.

230. The answer is A. *(Pritchard, ed 17. pp 281–282.)* The oxytocin challenge test is negative if the uterus contracts at least three times in a 10-minute interval, if each contraction lasts 40 seconds or longer, and if the contractions are not accompanied by a late deceleration of the fetal heart rate. Test results should be considered suspicious if late deceleration is uneven and unsustained in spite of continuing uterine contractions. In the presence of hyperstimulation of the uterus, judged either by the contraction frequency (more than one every 2 minutes) or length (longer than 90 seconds), late deceleration of the fetal heart rate may not signify uteroplacental disease.

231. The answer is D. *(Pritchard, ed 17. pp 222–223.)* The obstetric conjugate is the shortest distance between the promontory of the sacrum and the symphysis pubis. It generally measures 10.5 cm. Because the obstetric conjugate cannot be clinically measured, it is estimated by subtracting 1.5 to 2.0 cm from the diagonal conjugate, which is the distance from the lower margin of the symphysis to the sacral promontory. The true conjugate is measured from the top of the symphysis to the sacral promontory. The interspinous diameter is the transverse measurement of the midplane and generally is the smallest diameter of the pelvis.

232. The answer is C. *(Monif, ed 2. p 147.)* Spectinomycin is the treatment of choice for pregnant women who have an asymptomatic *Neisseria gonorrhoeae* infection and who are allergic to penicillin. Erythromycin is another drug effective in treating asymptomatic gonorrhea. Although tetracycline also is an effective alternative to penicillin, its use is contraindicated in pregnancy. Administration of chloramphenicol is not recommended to treat women, pregnant or not, who have cervical gonorrhea, and the use of ampicillin is contraindicated for penicillin-allergic patients.

233. The answer is E. *(Kase, p 1028.)* The synthetic sex steroids used in oral contraceptives may easily cross to the newborn in breast milk and cause jaundice in the newborn as well as other, as-yet-unrecognized effects. Other undesirable effects include suppression of lactation and increased risk of maternal thromboembolism in the early postpartum period. The pill has been associated with a decreased incidence of fibrocystic disease of the breast, but no association with breast cancer has been shown. Further, there is no known relationship to subsequent diabetes or an increase in thromboembolism in the newborn.

234. The answer is D. *(Pritchard, ed 17. pp 508–510.)* The ultrasonogram presented in the question clearly shows twins. The diagnosis can be made by noting the two heads (the circular densities). A hydatidiform mole would show no evidence of fetal parts or cranium. The presence of a spherical cranium rules out anencephaly. Because the placenta is anterior and superior, placenta previa is not present. Ultrasound has been very helpful in the diagnosis, early in gestation, of twins.

235. The answer is A. *(Pritchard, ed 17. pp 225–226.)* The anteroposterior diameter of the inlet of the anthropoid pelvis shown in the x-ray is greater than the transverse diameter. The anterior segment of an anthropoid pelvis is narrow, the ischial spines often are prominent, and the side walls may be somewhat convergent. In one American study, the anthropoid pelvis was found to be nearly twice as common (40 percent to 23 percent) in nonwhite women as in white women. This type of pelvis is far more likely than a gynecoid pelvis to be a source of dystocia.

236. The answer is E (all). *(Pritchard, ed 17. pp 345–347.)* Oxytocin is an octopeptide secreted by the neurohypophysis. Parenterally administered oxytocin stimulates uterine contractions and is widely used to induce and augment labor. Ergotrate and Methergine are alkaloid substances that are powerful stimulants of myometrial contractions. They are used after delivery to prevent and control postpartum hemorrhage but are too strong to use before delivery. Prostaglandin E_2 and F_2 are both capable of inducing and augmenting labor; however, in the United States neither is approved for use for these indications.

237. The answer is E (all). *(Sciarra, ed 51, vol 2, chap 29, pp 1–6.)* Normal resting uterine pressures are listed as less than 5 mmHg in the latent phase, less than 12 mmHg in the active phase, and less than 20 mmHg in the second stage of labor. Placental abruption, cephalopelvic disproportion, oxytocin (Pitocin) hyperstimulation, fetal malpresentation, and other conditions can cause elevated pressures.

238. The answer is C (2, 4). *(Pritchard, ed 17. p 260.)* Aspirin has been associated with platelet dysfunction and prolonged clotting times in both pregnant and nonpregnant individuals. Neonatal jaundice secondary to aspirin ingestion is caused by displacement of bilirubin from protein binding sites. The use of analgesic compounds that contain aspirin has also been associated with postdated gestations.

239. The answer is B (1, 3). *(Pritchard, ed 17. pp 273–274.)* $Rh_o(D)$ immune globulin (RhoGAM) is a concentrated sterile solution of human immunoglobulin G that contains anti-$Rh_o(D)$; it can prevent the formation of active $Rh_o(D)$ antibody in women, thereby impeding the development of Rh hemolytic disease of the newborn in subsequent deliveries. $Rh_o(D)$ immune globulin is usually given in an intramuscular dose of 300 μg within 72 hours of delivery. The failure rate, which is reported to be 1 to 2 percent, is attributed either to the development of sensitization in a subsequent pregnancy or to an unrecognized sensitization that already exists when the drug is administered. $Rh_o(D)$ immune globulin is of no benefit in ABO (blood group) incompatibility.

240. The answer is E (all). *(Pritchard, ed 17. p 251.)* The American College of Obstetricians and Gynecologists Task Force on Nutrition states that all the factors listed in the question as well as dieting, food fads, smoking, and hemoglobin levels less than 11 are associated with a poor nutritional state.

241. The answer is C (2, 4). *(Romney, ed 2. p 687.)* Edema is present to a greater or lesser degree in all pregnant women but most significantly among women who gain an excessive amount of weight. Edema of pregnancy has traditionally been treated with salt restriction and diuretics; however, it is now clear that sodium and water retention are normal processes during pregnancy. More water than sodium is retained, so unnecessary salt restriction and diuretics may cause intravascular depletion. Diuretics also may cause sodium and potassium depletion in the mother. Thiazide diuretics have been implicated in hemorrhagic pancreatitis and deterioration of glucose tolerance in the mother and in thrombocytopenia in the newborn. The best treatment of edema of pregnancy is bed rest in the lateral recumbent position, which should improve renal perfusion, and weight control if obesity is the major problem.

242. The answer is E (all). *(Pritchard, ed 17. p 708.)* Prolonged or rapid labor, oxytocin stimulation of labor, and twin pregnancy all predispose to uterine atony and, thus, to postpartum hemorrhage. A uterus that has required oxytocin in order to provide adequate labor is likely to need large amounts of oxytocin afterwards in order to stay contracted. A uterus that has stretched to accommodate twin gestations is likely to be atonic after it is emptied. No explanation is given for the clinical finding that a uterus that has been hypertonic and yielded a rapid labor is predisposed to atony.

243. The answer is C (2, 4). *(Pritchard, ed 17. p 475.)* Of the several methods to treat cervical incompetence, the McDonald and the Shirodkar cerclages are the two most commonly performed. The McDonald cerclage is accomplished by inserting a nonabsorbable suture in a purse-string fashion as high on the cervix as possible. With the Shirodkar cerclage the vaginal mucosa is incised anteriorly and posteriorly and the nonabsorbable suture is placed submucosally to encircle the cervix. Of the two procedures, the McDonald technique is easier and causes less scarring. Success rates of both procedures are 85 to 90 percent.

244. The answer is D (4). *(Pritchard, ed 17. pp 870–871.)* Guidelines from the American College of Obstetricians and Gynecologists state that a patient with a prior low transverse cesarean section may attempt a vaginal delivery following informed consent of the risks involved. Although the issue of prior cesarean section for CPD is controversial, this prior procedure is not an absolute contraindication for a trial of labor. A classic incision is a contraindication because of a high risk of uterine rupture. X-ray pelvimetry is not required prior to a trial of labor. Also, a prior vaginal delivery is not necessary.

245. The answer is D (4.) *(Pritchard, ed 17. p 282.)* The oxytocin challenge test assesses the ability of the fetoplacental unit to withstand the stress of labor. After external monitors have measured the baseline activity of the uterus and fetal heart for 10 minutes, intravenous oxytocin is infused at a rate of 0.5 mU/minute. The rate is doubled every 15 to 20 minutes until three contractions, each of which lasts for 40 to 60 seconds, occur every 10 minutes. The test is considered positive if fetal heart rate consistently decelerates once uterine contractions have begun.

246. The answer is E (all). *(Pritchard, ed 17. p 737.)* Uterine hemorrhage after the first postpartum week is most often the result of retained placental fragments or subinvolution of the placental site. Curettage may do more harm than benefit by stimulating increased bleeding. Initial therapy should be aimed at decreasing the bleeding by stimulating uterine contractions with the use of Pitocin, Methergine, or Ergotrate. Prostaglandins could also be used in this setting.

247. The answer is E (all). *(Pritchard, ed 17. p 361.)* Hypotension can result following sympathetic blockade from the anesthetic agent. Bladder distention usually due to blocking of the sensory fibers from the bladder can also be seen. Headaches result from persistent leakage of cerebrospinal fluid, which in the case of an epidural is the result of an inadvertent arachnoid puncture. Finally, the hypertensive response to Methergine or Ergotrate is most commonly seen when conduction anesthesia has been used.

248. The answer is A (1, 2, 3). *(Pritchard, ed 17. pp 286–287.)* The types of uniform decelerations are generally described. Early decelerations (type I) are usually a benign pattern attributed to head compression. Late decelerations (type II) are often an ominous pattern indicating uteroplacental insufficiency causing fetal hypoxia. Persistent tachycardia may indicate a fetal response to hypoxia and compromise. Variable decelerations (type III) are not related to contractions and are usually associated with cord compression. Tachycardia is associated with febrile illness and, more rarely, fetal thyrotoxicosis. Beat-to-beat variability refers to the normal variation in time interval between successive *r* waves in the fetal ECG. Loss of beat-to-beat variability may also be indicative of fetal compromise.

249. The answer is B (1, 3). *(Monif, ed 2. pp 18–26.)* Tetracycline may cause fetal dental anomalies and inhibition of bone growth if administered during the second trimester, and it is a potential teratogen to first-trimester fetuses. Tetracycline administration also can cause severe hepatic decompensation in the mother, especially during the third trimester. Chloramphenicol may cause the ''gray baby'' syndrome (symptoms of which include vomiting, impaired respiration, hypothermia, and, finally, cardiovascular collapse) in neonates who have received large doses of the drug. No notable adverse effects have been associated with the use of penicillin or ampicillin.

250–254. The answers are: 250-C, 251-E, 252-A, 253-E, 254-B. *(Pritchard, ed 17. pp 259–260.)* The recommendations concerning immunization during pregnancy offered by the American College of Obstetricians and Gynecologists are as follows:

1. Administration of influenza vaccine is recommended if the underlying disease is serious.

2. Typhoid immunization is recommended when traveling to an endemic region.

3. Hepatitis A immunization is recommended after exposure or before travel to developing countries.

4. Cholera immunization should be given only to meet travel requirements.

5. Tetanus-diphtheria immunization should be given if a primary series has never been administered or if 10 years have elapsed without receiving a booster.

6. Immunization for poliomyelitis is mandatory during an epidemic but otherwise not recommended.

7. Smallpox immunization is unnecessary since the disease has been eradicated.

8. Immunization for yellow fever is recommended before travel to a high-risk area.

9. Mumps and rubella immunizations are contraindicated.

10. Administration of rabies vaccine is unaffected by pregnancy.

ABNORMALITIES OF PREGNANCY

Spontaneous Abortion, Ectopic Pregnancies, and Trophoblastic Disease

DIRECTIONS: Each question below contains five suggested responses. Select the **one best** response to each question.

255. The karyotype of a complete hydatidiform mole is

(A) 46,XY
(B) 45,X
(C) 46,XX
(D) 69,XXX
(E) none of the above

256. Undesirable side effects of hypertonic saline induction of abortion include all the following EXCEPT

(A) hyperosmolar crisis
(B) disseminated intravascular coagulation
(C) bleeding
(D) birth of a live fetus
(E) myometrial necrosis

Questions 257–259

A 19-year-old primigravid woman is expecting her first child; she is 12 weeks pregnant by dates. She has vaginal bleeding and an enlarged-for-dates uterus. In addition, no fetal heart sounds are heard. An ultrasound is obtained, as shown on the next page.

257. The most likely diagnosis of this woman's condition is

(A) sarcoma botryoides
(B) tuberculous endometritis
(C) adenocarcinoma of the uterus
(D) hydatidiform mole
(E) normal pregnancy

258. The safest and most reliable method for early diagnosis of this woman's condition is

(A) amniography
(B) ultrasonography
(C) abdominal roentgenogram
(D) pelvic arteriography
(E) human chorionic gonadotropin (HCG) titer

259. After uterine evacuation, management of the woman described above, who has no clinical or radiographic evidence of metastatic disease, should include

(A) weekly HCG titers
(B) hysterectomy
(C) single-agent chemotherapy
(D) combination chemotherapy
(E) radiation therapy

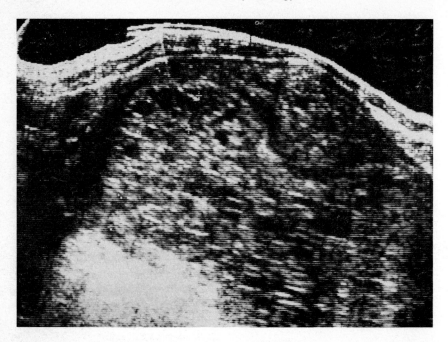

260. The most frequent pathogen currently implicated in infectious causes of early abortion is

(A) *Brucella abortus*
(B) *Listeria monocytogenes*
(C) *Toxoplasma gondii*
(D) *Mycoplasma hominis*
(E) *Streptococcus agalacture*

261. After an initial pregnancy resulted in a spontaneous loss in the first trimester, your patient is concerned about the possibility of this recurring. An appropriate answer to her would be that the chance of recurrence

(A) depends on the genetic makeup of the prior abortus
(B) is no different than it was prior to her miscarriage
(C) is increased to approximately 50 percent
(D) is increased most likely to greater than 50 percent
(E) depends on the sex of the prior abortus

262. Rates of successful pregnancy following three spontaneous losses (habitual abortion) are

(A) very poor
(B) slightly worse than those in the baseline population
(C) no different from those in the baseline population
(D) just under 50 percent
(E) good unless cervical incompetence is diagnosed

263. Spontaneous abortion and resorption in tubal pregnancies

(A) are uncommon
(B) are usually seen with isthmic implantations
(C) result in complete healing of the fallopian tube
(D) are usually seen with ampullary implantations
(E) require surgical intervention

264. All the following statements concerning chromosomal aberrations in abortions are true EXCEPT

(A) 45,X is more prevalent in chromosomally abnormal term babies than in abortus products
(B) approximately 50 percent of spontaneous abortions have chromosomal abnormalities
(C) trisomy 16 is the most common trisomy in abortuses
(D) despite the relatively high frequency of Down syndrome at term, most Down fetuses will abort spontaneously
(E) stillbirths have ten times the incidence of chromosomal abnormalities as live births

265. Which of the following findings is most commonly associated with ectopic pregnancy?

(A) Abnormal menstrual history
(B) Negative urine pregnancy test
(C) Abdominal pain
(D) Positive test for the beta subunit of human chorionic gonadotropin
(E) Adnexal mass on pelvic examination or sonography

266. A 32-year-old woman, gravida 3, para 3, presents with abdominal pain. Her last menstrual period was 6 weeks ago, and a pregnancy test is positive. The specimen shown below is obtained at laparotomy. The most likely diagnosis is

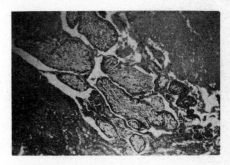

(A) incomplete abortion
(B) missed abortion
(C) hydatidiform mole
(D) tubal ectopic pregnancy
(E) none of the above

267. A 19-year-old woman comes to the emergency room and reports that she had passed out at work earlier in the day. She has mild vaginal bleeding, and her abdomen is diffusely tender and distended. In addition, she complains of shoulder and abdominal pain. Her temperature is 36.4°C (97.6°F); pulse rate, 120 per minute; and blood pressure, 96/50 mmHg. To confirm the diagnosis suggested by the available clinical data, which of the following diagnostic procedures would best be utilized?

(A) A pregnancy test
(B) Posterior colpotomy
(C) Dilatation and curettage
(D) Culdocentesis
(E) Laparoscopy

268. Which of the following statements concerning abdominal pregnancy is correct?

(A) Gastrointestinal symptoms are quite often severe
(B) Fetal survival is approximately 50 percent
(C) Aggressive attempts should be made to remove the placenta at the time of initial surgery
(D) It may result in infectious morbidity prior to the diagnosis
(E) It is usually the result of a primary abdominal implantation

269. Which of the following statements correctly applies to ectopic pregnancy?

(A) The Arias-Stella reaction is diagnostic of ectopic pregnancy
(B) Interstitial ectopic pregnancies generally rupture later, bleed more severely, and are usually more difficult to diagnose than isthmic or ampullary pregnancies
(C) Isthmic ectopic pregnancies are the most common
(D) Most ectopic pregnancies can be diagnosed sonographically by detecting a fetal sac in the adnexal region, outside the uterine cavity
(E) Tubal abortions do not cause significant intraperitoneal hemorrhage

DIRECTIONS: Each question below contains four suggested responses of which **one or more** is correct. Select

A	if	**1, 2, and 3**	are correct
B	if	**1 and 3**	are correct
C	if	**2 and 4**	are correct
D	if	**4**	is correct
E	if	**1, 2, 3, and 4**	are correct

270. Indications for instituting single-agent chemotherapy following evacuation of a hydatidiform mole usually include

(1) a rise in HCG titers
(2) a plateau of HCG titers for 3 successive weeks
(3) failure of HCG titers to return to normal 8 weeks after evacuation
(4) appearance of liver or brain metastases

271. Signs helpful in differentiating a tubal pregnancy from a pelvic infection include which of the following?

(1) High fever
(2) Enlarged uterus
(3) Presence of beta HCG
(4) Leukocytosis

272. Criteria that are especially reliable in determining a patient's response to chemotherapy for gestational trophoblastic disease include

(1) duration of the disease
(2) urine levels of HCG
(3) sites of metastases
(4) the patient's age

273. Observations on the role of actinomycin D and methotrexate in the management of gestational trophoblastic disease suggest that

(1) resistance to one agent results in cross-resistance to the other
(2) actinomycin D is safer than methotrexate for women whose liver function is impaired
(3) there is no additive effect in combining the two agents
(4) actinomycin D is as effective as methotrexate for primary treatment

274. Determination of the presence of a growing tumor in a patient who has gestational trophoblastic disease could be established by

(1) serial chest x-rays
(2) evaluation of menstrual function
(3) presence of lactation
(4) serial HCG titers

Spontaneous Abortion, Ectopic Pregnancies, and Trophoblastic Disease

Answers

255. The answer is C. *(Pritchard, ed 17. p 446.)* A hydatidiform mole is the transformation of the placenta into grapelike cysts with poorly vascularized and edematous villi and trophoblastic proliferation. The karyotype of a complete hydatidiform mole is believed to derive from a paternal haploid that duplicates to the 46,XX status. Partial moles with a concomitant fetus are often triploid (69,XXX or 69,XXY).

256. The answer is D. *(Pritchard, ed 17. pp 482–483.)* The birth of a live fetus is seen when prostaglandins are used to induce abortions. Intravascular injection of hypertonic saline can result in a hyperosmolar state as well as disseminated intravascular coagulation. Intrauterine injection can result in myometrial necrosis.

257. The answer is D. *(Jeanty, pp 213–215. Romney, ed 2. pp 1094–1097.)* The history, clinical picture, and a tissue sample of the woman described in the question are characteristic of hydatidiform mole. The most common initial symptoms include an enlarged-for-dates uterus and continuous or intermittent bleeding in the first two trimesters. Other symptoms include hypertension, proteinuria, and hyperthyroidism. Hydatidiform mole is ten times as common in the Far East as in North America, and it occurs more frequently in women over 45 years of age. A tissue sample would show a villus with hydropic changes and no vessels. Grossly, these lesions appear as small, clear clusters of grapelike vesicles, the passage of which confirms the diagnosis.

258. The answer is B. *(Sciarra, ed 51, vol 4, chap 48, pp 1–27.)* Ultrasonography is the safest and the most reliable method for early diagnosis of hydatidiform mole. Amniography, although another accurate method, requires percutaneous insertion of a needle into the uterine cavity and injection of a radiopaque contrast dye, which carries a risk of radiation exposure to a normal fetus. An abdominal roentgenogram cannot demonstrate a hydatidiform mole; however, if a fetal skeleton is visualized, it is unlikely that a hydatidiform mole also exists since coexisting molar and fetal pregnancies are rare. Elevated human chorionic gonadotropin (HCG) titers are not diagnostic. Pelvic arteriography would expose an accompanying normal fetus to high doses of radiation.

259. The answer is A. *(Sciarra, ed 51, vol 4, chap 48, pp 1–27.)* The condition of women who have hydatidiform moles but no evidence of metastatic disease should be followed routinely after uterine evacuation by HCG titers. Most authorities agree that prophylactic chemotherapy should not be employed in the routine management of women having hydatidiform moles, because 85 to 90 percent of affected patients will require no further treatment. For a young woman in whom preservation of reproductive function is important, surgery is not routinely indicated.

260. The answer is D. *(Pritchard, ed 17. pp 469–470.)* There have been increased investigations linking *Mycoplasma* infections with early abortions. There may be a role for preconceptual tetracycline therapy in couples with histories of habitual abortions. However, tetracycline agents are not generally considered appropriate in pregnancy.

261. The answer is B. *(Pritchard, ed 17. p 474.)* An initial spontaneous abortion, irrespective of the karyotype or sex of the child, does not change the risk for having a recurrence in a future pregnancy. The rate is commonly quoted as 15 percent of all known pregnancies.

262. The answer is B. *(Pritchard, ed 17. pp 474–475.)* A variety of therapies have resulted in successful pregnancy rates of 70 to 85 percent following a diagnosis of habitual abortion. When cervical incompetence is present and a cerclage is placed, success rates range as high as 90 percent.

263. The answer is D. *(Pritchard, ed 17. pp 424–425.)* Ectopic pregnancies spontaneously abort and resorb in up to 50 percent of tubal pregnancies. They are more common with ampullary implants, while isthmic insertions usually rupture through the fallopian tube. Sequelae of the tubal abortion include a hematosalpinx and placental polyps within the endosalpinx.

264. The answer is A. *(Thompson, ed 4. pp 126–128.)* Chromosomal abnormalities are found in approximately 50 percent of spontaneous abortions, 5 percent of stillbirths, and 0.5 percent of live born babies. In the spontaneous losses, trisomy 16 is the most common trisomy with 45,X the most common single abnormality found. At term, trisomy 16 is rarely seen and 45,X is seen in approximately 1 in 20,000 births. It is estimated that 99 percent of 45,X and 75 percent of trisomy 21 conceptuses are lost before term.

265. The answer is D. *(Pritchard, ed 17. pp 423–438.)* All the findings listed in the question may be associated with extrauterine pregnancy, but the extremely sensitive radioimmunoassay for the beta subunit of human chorionic gonadotropin is so sensitive that it is virtually always positive in these cases. Unfortunately, this test is *not* diagnostic of the condition.

266. The answer is D. *(Sciarra, ed 51, vol 6, chap 29, pp 1–6.)* The photomicrograph accompanying the question shows villi within a tubular structure; the villi are easily identified by the presence of cytotrophoblasts. The diagnosis is tubal ectopic pregnancy. Molar pregnancy, incomplete abortion, and missed abortion also can be associated with the presence of villi, but specimens from these disorders would not be obtained at laparotomy.

267. The answer is D. *(Kistner, ed 4, pp 268–277.)* The clinical history presented in this question is a classic one for a ruptured tubal pregnancy accompanied by hemoperitoneum. Because pregnancy tests are negative in almost 50 percent of cases, they are of little practical value in an emergency. Dilatation and curettage would not permit rapid enough diagnosis, and the results obtained by this procedure are variable. Posterior colpotomy requires an operating room, surgical anesthesia, and an experienced operator with a scrubbed and gowned associate. Refined optic and electronic systems have improved the accuracy of laparoscopy, but this new equipment is not always available, and the procedure requires an operating room and, usually, surgical anesthesia. Culdocentesis is a rapid, nonsurgical method to confirm the presence of unclotted, intraabdominal blood from a ruptured tubal pregnancy.

268. The answer is D. *(Pritchard, ed 17. pp 433–436.)* Abdominal pregnancy usually follows a tubal pregnancy with either tubal rupture or spontaneous passage through the fimbriated end. Although women with abdominal pregnancy usually report an increase in gastrointestinal symptoms, these are rarely severe enough to lead to investigation. Fetal death rates are reported to be above 90 percent with abdominal pregnancies. Infection of the gestational products can occur especially when the placenta adheres to the intestines. This can lead to abscess formation and the possibility of rupture. Although leaving the placenta in the abdomen following surgical delivery predisposes to postoperative coagulation problems as well as the need for subsequent surgery, these complications can be less severe than the hemorrhage associated with attempts at removal at the time of primary delivery. If the placenta cannot easily be removed, recommendations are to leave it in place at the time of the first surgery.

269. The answer is B. *(Pritchard, ed 17. pp 423–438.)* Ectopic pregnancies most commonly occur in the ampullary portion of the fallopian tube. When they do occur in the interstitial portion of the tube (2.5 percent of cases), they are harder to diagnose, may rupture late because of the thick myometrium into which they grow, and often lead to severe, life-threatening hemorrhage because of the tremendous vascularity of the area. The histologic finding of an Arias-Stella reaction suggests abnormal pregnancy but is *not* diagnostic of ectopic gestation. Ultrasound examination is most useful in indirectly ruling out ectopic pregnancy by demonstrating an intrauterine gestation, as coexistence of a second ectopic pregnancy is extremely rare. Even tubal abortion can lead to severe intraperitoneal bleeding.

270. The answer is A (1, 2, 3). *(Romney, ed 2. pp 1098–1099.)* Single-agent chemotherapy usually is instituted if levels of HCG have remained elevated 8 weeks after evacuation of a hydatidiform mole. Approximately 50 percent of the patients who have persistently high HCG titers will develop malignant sequelae. If HCG titers rise or reach a plateau for 2 to 3 successive weeks following molar evacuation, a single-agent chemotherapy should be instituted, provided that the trophoblastic disease has not metastasized to the liver or brain. The presence of such metastases usually requires initiation of combination chemotherapy.

271. The answer is A (1, 2, 3). *(Pritchard, ed 17. p 429.)* Although ectopics can present with a low-grade febrile response, temperatures above 38°C are unusual with ectopic pregnancies. Because of placental hormone production from the ectopic pregnancy, the uterus will soften and enlarge during the first 3 months of pregnancy, and assays for beta HCG will be positive. Approximately one half of ectopic pregnancies will have an elevated white count up to a maximum of about 30,000. However, leukocytosis is not a sensitive test to separate ectopic pregnancy from pelvic infection.

272. The answer is A (1, 2, 3). *(DiSaia, ed 2. p 196.)* Women who have had gestational trophoblastic disease for less than 4 months, whose 24-hour urine titers of HCG are less than 100,000 IU, and whose metastases are limited to the vagina or lungs have a 95-percent cure rate and are thus considered low-risk patients. Patients whose disease has lasted for more than 4 months, whose HCG titer is greater than 100,000 IU per 24 hours, and who have liver or brain metastases, on the other hand, are classified as high-risk patients.

273. The answer is C (2, 4). *(DiSaia, ed 2. pp 200–211.)* The first successful treatment regimen for women who had gestational trophoblastic disease consisted of single-agent methotrexate chemotherapy. Subsequent studies combining methotrexate, actinomycin D, and an alkylating agent were successful in treating methotrexate-resistant trophoblastic disease. Actinomycin D, then studied as a single agent, proved to be as effective as methotrexate; in addition, it was not hampered by cross-resistance in methotrexate-resistant tumors and was safer to use in women who had impaired liver function.

274. The answer is D (4). *(Romney, ed 2. pp 1093–1094.)* Viable trophoblastic tissue produces HCG; therefore, the presence of elevated HCG titers confirms the amount of functioning trophoblastic tissue and thus the size of the tumor. Monitoring serial HCG titers allows the physician to determine not only the need for chemotherapy but also its effectiveness. Theca-lutein cysts tend to decrease in size following evacuation of a hydatidiform mole despite the persistence of viable trophoblastic cells; and normal cyclic menstruation may reappear in spite of continued disease activity. Chest x-ray changes often persist for several months after HCG titers have returned to normal.

Medical, Surgical, and Obstetrical Complications of Pregnancy

DIRECTIONS: Each question below contains five suggested responses. Select the **one best** response to each question.

275. Which of the following statements concerning the use of magnesium sulfate in pregnancy is true?

(A) Magnesium sulfate is an effective antihypertensive agent when used at serum levels to prevent convulsions
(B) A therapeutic range of 7 to 10 mEq/L is necessary to prevent convulsions
(C) An intramuscular regimen of magnesium sulfate can result in therapeutic levels as effectively as continuous IV infusion
(D) Magnesium will not enter the fetal circulation
(E) Monitoring the presence of the patellar reflex is a poor indicator of magnesium sulfate levels

276. All the following may contribute to a diagnosis of severe pregnancy-induced hypertension EXCEPT

(A) 24-hour urine protein of 3500 mg
(B) platelet count of less than 100,000/ml^3
(C) burr cells and schistocytes on a peripheral smear
(D) elevated SGOT
(E) epigastric pain

277. A 24-year-old woman appears at 8 weeks of pregnancy and reveals a history of pulmonary embolism 7 years ago during her first pregnancy. She was treated with intravenous heparin followed by several months of oral warfarin (Coumadin) and has had no further evidence of thromboembolic disease for over 6 years. Which of the following statements about her current condition is true?

(A) Having no evidence of disease for over 5 years means that her risk of thromboembolism is not greater than normal
(B) Impedance plethysmography is not a useful study to evaluate her for deep venous thrombosis in pregnancy
(C) Doppler ultrasonography is not a useful technique to evaluate her for deep venous thrombosis in pregnancy
(D) The patient should be placed on low-dose heparin therapy throughout her pregnancy and the puerperium
(E) She is at highest risk for recurrent thromboembolism during the second trimester of pregnancy

Questions 278–280

A 24-year-old primigravid woman develops spider angiomata, palmar erythema, and diffuse pruritus at 28 weeks gestation. You obtain a set of liver function tests, which reveal the following serum levels: alkaline phosphatase, 190 IU/L (normal: 21 to 91 IU/L); glutamic oxaloacetic transaminase, 38 IU/L (normal: 6 to 18 IU/L); total bilirubin, 1.8 mg/100 ml (normal: 0.3 to 1.0 mg/100 ml); direct bilirubin, 1.0 mg/100 ml (normal: 0.1 to 0.3 mg/100 ml).

278. What is the most likely diagnosis of this woman's condition?

(A) Cirrhosis
(B) Infectious hepatitis
(C) Cholestasis
(D) Acute pancreatitis
(E) Cholecystitis

279. The most appropriate treatment would be

(A) observation
(B) bed rest and high-protein diet
(C) oral corticosteroids
(D) low-fat diet
(E) oral cholestyramine

280. After delivery, the physician should advise the woman to

(A) avoid further pregnancies
(B) avoid high-fat foods
(C) avoid oral contraceptives
(D) have a cholecystectomy
(E) none of the above

281. All the following statements about autoimmune thrombocytopenic purpura (ATP) in pregnancy are true EXCEPT that

(A) platelet production is normal or greater in the bone marrow
(B) bleeding time may be normal because of the presence in the circulation of young, hyperactive platelets
(C) peripheral destruction of antibody-coated circulating platelets may result in abnormally low maternal platelet counts
(D) cesarean section may not always prevent fetal hemorrhage
(E) a maternal platelet count about 100,000/mm³ at the time of delivery ensures safety for the newborn

282. The initial maternal immunological response to a primary rubella infection is the elaboration of

(A) immunoglobulin M
(B) immunoglobulin G
(C) immunoglobulin A
(D) immunoglobulin D
(E) complement-fixation antibodies

283. Which of the following statements is true about placental abruption?

(A) Coagulopathy results from the consumption of clotting factors by the tetroplacental clot
(B) More than 50 percent of patients with this condition develop significant hypofibrinogenemia (less than 150 mg/dl)
(C) Less than 10 percent of patients with this condition develop significant hypofibrinogenemia (less than 150 mg/dl)
(D) Vigorous fluid, blood, and electrolyte replacement is generally adequate to prevent severe renal failure
(E) Many patients require dialysis despite vigorous fluid, blood, and electrolyte replacement

284. Which of the following statements concerning placenta previa is true?

(A) Its incidence decreases with maternal age
(B) Its incidence is unaffected by parity
(C) The initial hemorrhage is painless and rarely fatal
(D) Management no longer includes a "double set-up"
(E) Bleeding is usually painful

285. Which of the following statements about placenta previa is true?

(A) Consumptive coagulopathy is a frequent complication
(B) The first episode of hemorrhage is generally severe enough to warrant immediate delivery
(C) Most cases of placenta previa diagnosed sonographically at the 22d week of gestation will never present as clinical problems
(D) Abdominal delivery is contraindicated if the fetus is dead
(E) With modern techniques, "double set-up examination" is an obsolete procedure

286. Viremia and the presence of rubella virus in the throat of infected individuals bear which of the following relationships to the onset of the rubella rash?

(A) They precede the rash by 5 to 7 days
(B) They precede the rash by 1 to 2 days
(C) They occur coincidentally with the rash
(D) They occur 1 to 2 days after the rash
(E) They bear no consistent relationship to the onset of the rash

287. For patients developing preeclampsia in their first pregnancy, which of the following is an associated future risk?

(A) Diabetes mellitus
(B) Chronic hypertension
(C) Habitual abortion
(D) Chronic liver disease
(E) Increased risk of third trimester stillborns in subsequent pregnancies

288. Although rheumatic heart disease is becoming less common, it still occurs during pregnancy. Deteriorating cardiac status in a pregnant woman is most likely to be associated with

(A) aortic regurgitation
(B) aortic stenosis
(C) mitral regurgitation
(D) mitral stenosis
(E) tricuspid regurgitation

289. All the following statements regarding drugs used in the treatment of tuberculosis are true EXCEPT

(A) rifampin may cause a flu-like syndrome
(B) patients receiving INH may develop a peripheral neuropathy
(C) patients receiving INH may develop optic neuritis
(D) ototoxicity is a side effect of streptomycin
(E) a positive antinuclear antibody (ANA) titer may be seen with INH therapy

290. All the following statements concerning polyhydramnios are true EXCEPT

(A) therapeutic amniocentesis is performed only to relieve maternal distress
(B) the incidence of major malformations in the presence of polyhydramnios is 20 percent
(C) diuretics and salt and water restriction are effective and safe treatment options
(D) placental abruption, uterine dysfunction, and postpartum hemorrhage occur more frequently in the presence of polyhydramnios
(E) the rapid removal of fluid is contraindicated

291. Frequency, urgency, dysuria, and pyuria without bacteriuria may be the consequence of urethritis caused by

(A) *Escherichia coli*
(B) group B streptococci
(C) *Chlamydiae trachomatis*
(D) coagulase-negative staphylococci
(E) none of the above

292. Which of the following statements concerning urinary tract infections in pregnancy is true?

(A) In cases of acute pyelonephritis, the most common organism cultured is group B streptococcus
(B) Women with sickle cell trait possess a protective mechanism against urinary tract infections, and they have an overall lower incidence of bacteriuria during pregnancy
(C) Culture of a clean-voided, midstream urine specimen is adequate for the diagnosis of asymptomatic bacteriuria
(D) Because as many as 40 percent of women with asymptomatic bacteriuria may progress to symptomatic disease, intravenous antibiotic therapy should be instituted once the diagnosis is made
(E) None of the above

293. Which of the following statements concerning hepatitis infection in pregnancy is true?

(A) Hepatitis B core antigen status is the most sensitive indicator of positive vertical transmission of disease

(B) Hepatitis B is the most common form of hepatitis after blood transfusion

(C) The proper treatment of infants born to infected mothers includes the administration of hepatitis B immune globulin, as well as Heptavax-B

(D) Patients who develop chronic active hepatitis should undergo therapeutic abortion

(E) None of the above

DIRECTIONS: Each question below contains four suggested responses of which **one or more** is correct. Select

A	if	**1, 2, and 3**	are correct
B	if	**1 and 3**	are correct
C	if	**2 and 4**	are correct
D	if	**4**	is correct
E	if	**1, 2, 3, and 4**	are correct

294. True statements concerning infants born to mothers with active tuberculosis include which of the following?

(1) The risk of active disease during the first year of life may approach 50 percent if untreated
(2) BCG vaccination of the newborn infant without evidence of active disease is an appropriate form of therapy
(3) Future ability for tuberculin skin testing is lost after BCG administration to the newborn
(4) Neonatal infection is most likely acquired by aspiration of infected amniotic fluid

295. True statements concerning AIDS and pregnancy include which of the following?

(1) The rate of perinatal transmission of HTLV-III/LAV from infected pregnant women is unknown, but is probably low
(2) There is no need to delay the onset of pregnancy in women who are HTLV-III/LAV antibody positive, but show no manifestation of the disease
(3) Cesarean section delivery has been shown to be of benefit in preventing perinatal transmission of HTLV-III/LAV
(4) Infected women should be advised against breastfeeding to avoid postnatal transmission

296. Women who have systemic lupus erythematosus should be counseled that

(1) pregnancy is contraindicated, because it will exacerbate the disease
(2) if pregnant, they should have a therapeutic abortion to prevent a progression of their symptoms
(3) their disease is likely to inhibit their fertility
(4) their disease is likely to flare up after delivery

SUMMARY OF DIRECTIONS

A	B	C	D	E
1,2,3 only	1,3 only	2,4 only	4 only	All are correct

297. True statements concerning vaccines include

(1) inactivated vaccines are probably not hazardous to either the mother or the fetus
(2) no cases of congenital rubella syndrome have been reported in fetuses born to mothers who were immunized early in pregnancy
(3) the polio virus has the ability to spread from the vaccine to susceptible individuals in the immediate environment
(4) nonimmune pregnant women who are exposed to children who recently received the MMR vaccine are at high risk of delivery of an infected fetus

298. True statements about hyperthyroidism in pregnancy include which of the following?

(1) Affected women may be treated with thiourea compounds
(2) It is harder to control in pregnant than in nonpregnant women
(3) It may cause neonatal thyrotoxicosis
(4) It is an indication for interrupting a pregnancy

299. Pregnant women who have diabetes mellitus are affected more often than nondiabetic women by which of the following conditions?

(1) Preeclampsia and eclampsia
(2) Infection
(3) Postpartum hemorrhage after vaginal delivery
(4) Hydramnios

300. Erythroblastosis fetalis can be caused by maternal incompatibility with which of the following fetal erythrocyte antigens?

(1) Kell
(2) Kidd
(3) Duffy
(4) Lewis

301. Pregnancy should be strongly discouraged in women who have

(1) atrial septal defect
(2) ventricular septal defect
(3) patent ductus arteriosus
(4) Eisenmenger's syndrome

302. Pregnancy has which of the following effects on diabetic women?

(1) Tendency toward ketoacidosis during early pregnancy
(2) Tendency toward hyperglycemia during early pregnancy
(3) Increase in insulin requirement during early pregnancy
(4) Increase in insulin requirement during late pregnancy

303. Hypothyroidism can be characterized by which of the following statements?

(1) It is uncommon during pregnancy
(2) It is associated with an increased abortion rate
(3) It is associated with an increased stillbirth rate
(4) It is generally improved by pregnancy

304. Ovarian neoplasms of pregnant women can be characterized by which of the following statements?

(1) They are usually malignant
(2) They are most often confined to one ovary
(3) They may spread transplacentally to the fetus
(4) They can be mistaken for a cystic corpus luteum

305. A 27-year-old woman (gravida 3, para 2) comes to the delivery floor at 37 weeks gestation. She has had no prenatal care. She complains that, on bending down to pick up her 2-year-old child, she experienced sudden, severe back pain. This pain now has persisted for 2 hours. Approximately 30 minutes ago she noted bright red blood coming from her vagina. By the time she arrives at the delivery floor, she is contracting strongly every 3 minutes; the uterus is quite firm even between contractions. By abdominal palpation the fetus is vertex with the head deeply engaged. Fetal heart rate is 130 beats per minute. The fundus is 38 cm above the symphysis. Blood for clotting is drawn, and a clot forms in 4 minutes. Clotting studies are sent to the laboratory. The initial course of action should probably include

(1) stabilizing maternal circulation
(2) administering oxytocin to stimulate labor
(3) inserting an intrauterine catheter for fetal monitoring
(4) administering heparin immediately

306. True statements about pregnancy-induced hypertension include which of the following?

(1) The incidence varies widely around the world
(2) Women who have had hypertension of pregnancy once have a 10 percent chance of developing it in a later pregnancy
(3) Elevations in systolic or diastolic blood pressures may be diagnostically significant even at blood pressure values less than 140/90 mmHg
(4) Young primiparous women have the lowest incidence

307. Premature separation of the placenta occurs more commonly than normal in association with which of the following conditions?

(1) Previous abruptio placentae
(2) Chronic hypertension
(3) Pregnancy-induced hypertension
(4) Delivery of twins

308. Nausea and vomiting are common in pregnancy. Hyperemesis gravidarum, however, is a much more serious and potentially fatal problem. Findings that should alert the physician to the diagnosis of hyperemesis gravidarum *early* in its course include

(1) electrocardiographic evidence of hypokalemia
(2) weight loss
(3) jaundice
(4) ketonuria

309. Common findings in the incompetent cervix syndrome include

(1) painless dilatation of the cervix
(2) a history of cervical trauma
(3) spontaneous rupture of the menbranes at midpregnancy
(4) recurrent miscarriage at 14 to 16 weeks gestation

DIRECTIONS: Each group of questions below consists of lettered headings followed by a set of numbered items. For each numbered item select the **one** lettered heading with which it is **most** closely associated. Each lettered heading may be used **once, more than once, or not at all.**

Questions 310–312

For each clinical situation that follows, select the most likely placental disorder.

(A) Placenta accreta
(B) Placenta circumvallata
(C) Placenta membranacea
(D) Placenta succenturiata
(E) Vasa praevia

310. A 24-year-old woman, gravida 2, para 1, goes into premature labor at 33 weeks gestation after an apparently normal antepartum course

311. An apparently normal pregnancy culminates in the spontaneous delivery of an infant who weighs 3.2 kg (7 lb) with Apgars 9/9. The placenta delivers spontaneously followed by an unusual amount of uterine bleeding

312. After the low forceps delivery of an infant who weighs 1.8 kg (4 lb) to a 27-year-old woman, gravida 4, para 3 (whose second baby was born by cesarean section owing to fetal distress but whose third baby delivered vaginally), the placenta does not deliver spontaneously. After 20 minutes the obstetrician attempts a manual removal but is unable to identify a plane of cleavage

Questions 313–316

For each description that follows, select the microorganism with which it is most likely to be associated.

(A) Rubella virus
(B) Cytomegalovirus
(C) Group A β-hemolytic streptococci
(D) Group B β-hemolytic streptococci
(E) *Toxoplasma gondii*

313. This organism may cause epidemics of puerperal sepsis

314. A pregnant woman may become infected with this organism by contact with infected cat feces

315. An effective vaccine exists for the prevention of adult infection with this organism

316. This organism is an important cause of neonatal sepsis and meningitis

Questions 317–321

For each description that follows, select the disorder with which it is most likely to be associated.

(A) Placental polyps
(B) Placenta previa
(C) Abruptio placentae
(D) Ectopic pregnancy
(E) Spontaneous abortion

317. Associated with the Arias-Stella phenomenon

318. Associated with premature placental separation

319. Associated with maternal hypertension

320. May be due to defective vascularization of the decidua caused by inflammation or atrophy

321. Usually accompanied by thickened placental villi, hemorrhage into the decidua basalis, and evidence of necrosis in tissues near the bleeding

Medical, Surgical, and Obstetrical Complications of Pregnancy

Answers

275. The answer is C. *(Pritchard, ed 17. pp 551–553.)* The appropriate use of $MgSO_4 \cdot 7H_2O$ will nearly always arrest eclamptic seizures and prevent recurrences. A therapeutic range of 4 to 7 mEq/L will prevent convulsions, and it can be achieved adequately and safely by either intravenous or intramuscular routes of administration after a loading dose of 10 g intramuscularly or 4 g intravenously. Maintenance is best achieved with a 2-g/hour continuous intravenous infusion or a 5-g intramuscular injection every 4 hours. Monitoring the presence or absence of the patellar reflex, which disappears at 10 mEq/L, is an accurate determination of the magnesium level. Respiratory arrest will occur at levels above 12 mEq/L. Magnesium ions will enter the fetal circulation, and they will equilibrate with maternal plasma levels. Magnesium sulfate in dosages used to prevent convulsions has no significant antihypertensive effect.

276. The answer is A. *(Pritchard, ed 17. pp 525–538.)* The diagnosis of severe pregnancy-induced hypertension is made from a combination of signs and symptoms. A diastolic blood pressure of greater than 100 mmHg, headaches, visual disturbances, and upper abdominal pain are all hallmarks of severe pregnancy-induced hypertension. Laboratory abnormalities seen in severe pregnancy-induced hypertension include an elevated SGOT, hyperbilirubinemia, thrombocytopenia, an evidence of microangiopathic hemolysis as seen by changes in the erythrocyte morphology, and elevated creatinine and uric acid levels.

277. The answer is D. *(Burrow, ed 2. pp 172–183.)* Patients with a history of thromboembolic disease in pregnancy are at high risk to develop it in subsequent pregnancies. Impedance plethysmography or Doppler ultrasonography are useful techniques even in pregnancy, and should be done as baseline studies. Patients should be treated prophylactically with low-dose heparin therapy through the postpartum period as this is the time of highest risk of this disease.

278–280. The answers are: 278-C, 279-E, 280-C. *(Pritchard, ed 17. pp 611–615.)* The most likely diagnosis for the woman described in the question is cholestatic jaundice of pregnancy (cholestasis). Spider angiomata and palmar erythema are normal occurrences in pregnant women and do not imply hepatic disease. Generalized pruritus in pregnancy, however, may be caused by cholestasis. In this disorder, bilirubin may or may not be elevated and elevation, if present, is usually mild. Although serum alkaline phosphatase levels may double during normal pregnancy, they are usually even higher in cholestasis of pregnancy. If placental (heat-stable) alkaline phosphatase can be distinguished from the hepatic isozyme, then hepatic alkaline phosphatase will show an increase in patients with cholestasis. Levels of serum glutamic-oxaloacetic transaminase may be mildly elevated.

The appropriate treatment for this condition, if the itching is intractable, is oral cholestyramine, an exchange resin that ties up bile salts in the gastrointestinal tract and presumably reduces their levels in the periphery. Although its safety in pregnancy is not unequivocally established, oral cholestyramine is commonly used for this condition when treatment is necessary.

Cholestasis tends to recur in subsequent pregnancies and to accompany use of oral contraceptives. If the patient is willing to go through another pregnancy with the symptoms described, pregnancy is not contraindicated; however, oral contraceptives are probably a poor choice for family planning in these patients. In the case described, there is no reason to suspect pancreatitis; cirrhosis is not exacerbated by pregnancy; the enzyme values do not support hepatitis; and the patient does not show symptoms of cholecystitis.

281. The answer is E. *(Burrow, ed 2. pp 74–76.)* ATP is an immunologic disorder wherein antibodies to an individual's own platelets lead to peripheral destruction of these cells by the reticuloendothelial system, thus leading to reduced numbers of circulating platelets. Platelets continue to be produced in greater than normal numbers, leading to large numbers of active young platelets in the circulation that may function to keep the bleeding time close to normal. Because maternal IgG antibody may cross the placenta, coating fetal platelets and leading to thrombocytopenia in the fetus, an atraumatic delivery should be accomplished to protect the fetus. Unfortunately, even cesarean section may not offer complete protection, as at least one case of neonatal hemorrhage and death following cesarean section has been reported. Maternal platelet counts above 100,000 do *not* guarantee adequate fetal counts.

282. The answer is A. *(Burrow, ed 2. p 337.)* The first response to a primary infection of rubella and other viruses is the elaboration of immunoglobulin M (IgM). Although IgM, once produced, is present for at least several weeks, rising levels of immunoglobulin G (IgG) account for the fact that IgG eventually constitutes nearly all antibody detected in the serum. Complement-fixation antibodies usually appear 7 to 10 days after appearance of the rubella rash.

283. The answer is D. *(Pritchard, ed 17. pp 398–401.)* Thirty percent of abruptions resulting in fetal death also result in significant hypofibrinogenemia. The mechanism of the coagulopathy is most likely *not* just the consumption of clotting factors by the retroplacental clot, but rather a disseminated intravascular coagulation. When severe hemorrhage occurs, there is definite risk of acute renal failure. This complication can be prevented through vigorous fluid, blood, and electrolyte replacement, thereby avoiding the need for dialysis.

284. The answer is C. *(Pritchard, ed 17. pp 410–411.)* The initial hemorrhage in placenta previa is usually painless and rarely fatal. If the fetus is premature and if hemorrhaging is not severe, vaginal examination of a woman suspected of having placenta previa frequently can be delayed until 37 weeks of gestation; this delay in the potentially hazardous examination reduces the risk of prematurity, which often is associated with placenta previa. Vaginal examination, when needed to determine whether a low-lying placenta is covering the internal os of the cervix, should be performed in an operating room fully prepared for an emergency cesarean section (i.e., a "double set-up"). Increasing maternal age and multiparity are associated with a higher incidence of placenta previa.

285. The answer is C. *(Pritchard, ed 17. pp 407–411.)* Unlike abruptio placentae, placenta previa is rarely complicated by coagulopathy. Most often the first episode of bleeding is relatively mild but should alert the physician to the possible diagnosis. Up to 45 percent of patients undergoing ultrasound examination in the second trimester may have low-lying placentas, but the majority of these migrate from the cervical os by the third trimester. Despite fetal loss, cesarean section may be needed to prevent further maternal hemorrhage. The double-setup examination still has a place in obstetrics.

286. The answer is A. *(Burrow, ed 2. p 335.)* Both viremia and the excretion of virus from the throats of individuals infected with rubella occur 5 to 7 days before the appearance of the characteristic maculopapular rash. The importance of this relationship is that by the time a pregnant woman first notes the appearance of a rash on one of her children, she already has been exposed to the disease and may, in fact, be infected. If one member of a family develops rubella, all other members who are susceptible to the disease usually become infected.

287. The answer is A. *(Pritchard, ed 17. pp 553–554.)* Careful long-term follow-up studies of preeclamptic women have failed to reveal long-term hypertensive disease. However, Chesley and colleagues showed diabetes to be 2.5 to 4 times more common in previously preeclamptic women than controls. When patients with chronic hypertension are removed from these studies, pure preeclampsia seems to have little other long-term risk.

288. The answer is D. *(Burrow, ed 2. pp 155–157.)* Nearly all the circulatory changes that normally accompany pregnancy are harmful to a woman who has mitral stenosis. Left atrial pressure rises because of increased cardiac output and shortened diastolic filling time; as a result, pulmonary flow is accentuated. Atrial fibrillation may occur suddenly during pregnancy, and pulmonary edema may supervene. Cardioversion may be necessary to reverse atrial fibrillation. Mitral regurgitation is unlikely to be worsened by pregnancy, although prophylaxis for subacute bacterial endocarditis would be indicated for affected women. Aortic stenosis is unusual as a pure lesion; associated problems, if they are going to develop at all, are most likely to develop in the immediate postpartum period, when rapid volume shifts can occur. Aortic regurgitation also is rare as pure lesion and again is most likely to cause problems just after delivery.

289. The answer is C. *(Burrow, ed 2. pp 422–423.)* Rifampin has occasionally been known to cause a flu-like syndrome, abdominal pain, acute renal failure, and thrombocytopenia. It may also resemble hepatitis and can cause orange urine, sweat, and tears. INH has been associated with hepatitis, hypersensitivity reactions, and peripheral neuropathies. The neuropathy can be prevented by the administration of pyridoxine, especially in the pregnant patient where pyridoxine requirements are increased. INH may also cause a rash, a fever, and a lupus-like syndrome with a positive ANA titer. Streptomycin has a potential for ototoxicity in both the mother and the fetus. The most commonly seen fetal side effects include minor vestibular impairment, auditory impairment, or both. Cases of severe and bilateral hearing loss and marked vestibular abnormalities have been reported with streptomycin use. Optic neuritis is a well-described side effect of ethambutol, although it is rare at the usual prescribed doses.

290. The answer is C. *(Pritchard, ed 17. pp 462–465.)* The occurrence of polyhydramnios is associated with an increase in perinatal mortality and a 20 percent incidence of major fetal malformations. A collection of greater than 3000 ml of fluid will usually cause symptoms. This occurs in 1 in 1000 singleton pregnancies. Maternal discomfort prior to term makes therapeutic amniocentesis necessary. Amniocentesis should be performed aseptically with the rate of withdrawal at 500 cc/hour in order to prevent premature labor and placental abruption. Dyspnea, pain, and inability to ambulate are all reasons for therapeutic amniocentesis. Salt restriction and diuretics offer no effective results, and they may pose dangers to the patient.

291. The answer is C. *(Wilson, ed 7. p 580.)* Frequency and urgency, as well as dysuria, especially at the time of voiding, are all typical symptoms of cystitis. White blood cells and possibly red blood cells are seen, along with bacteria, on microscopic examination. *Chlamydiae trachomatis*, a common pathogen of the genitourinary tract, should be suspected in the presence of symptoms of cystitis, but no bacteria on urinalysis.

292. The answer is C. *(Pritchard, ed 17. pp 580–583.)* Asymptomatic bacteriuria is present in approximately 5 percent of all pregnant women at their first prenatal visit. The overall incidence varies between 2 and 12 percent, depending on the patient population. The highest incidence appears to be in black, multiparous women of low socioeconomic status who have sickle cell trait. Significant bacteriuria is required for diagnosis, which is accomplished by culturing a clean-catch, midstream, voided specimen and demonstrating positive bacterial growth. This avoids routine catheterization with its subsequent increased risk of infection. Twenty to forty percent of women with asymptomatic bacteriuria will progress to a symptomatic infection. Therefore, treatment should be instigated after the diagnosis is made. However, outpatient oral management is appropriate with asymptomatic or symptomatic bacteriuria of the lower urinary tract.

293. The answer is C. *(Pritchard, ed 17. pp 614–615.)* Persons at increased risk for hepatitis B infection include homosexuals, IV drug abusers, health care personnel, and individuals who have received blood or blood products. Hepatitis B is also endemic in some populations of Asia and Africa. The mode of transmission for hepatitis B is through blood and blood products, as well as saliva, vaginal secretions, and semen. However, because of intensive screening of blood for type B hepatitis, non-A,non-B hepatitis has become the major form of hepatitis after blood transfusion. Venereal transmission and the sharing of needles in persons who are IV drug abusers have had major roles in the transmission of hepatitis B. A variety of immunologic markers exist to identify patients who either have active disease, are chronic carriers of disease, or have antibody protection. Among the markers, the e antigen is very similar to the virus and is an indicator of the infectious state. Mothers who are e antigen positive are more likely to transmit the disease to their infants, whereas the absence of the e antigen in the presence of e antibody appears to be protective. Chronic active hepatitis does not necessarily warrant therapeutic abortion. Fertility is decreased, but pregnancy may proceed on a normal course, as long as steroid therapy is continued. Prematurity and fetal loss are increased, but there is no increase in malformations.

294. The answer is A (1, 2, 3). *(Burrow, ed 2. pp 422–423.)* The goal of management in the infant born to a mother with active tuberculosis is preventing early neonatal infection. Congenital infection, acquired either by a hematogenous route or by aspiration of infected amniotic fluid, is rare. Most neonatal infection is acquired by postpartum maternal contact. The risk of active disease during the first year of life may approach 50 percent if prophylaxis is not instituted. BCG vaccination and daily INH (isonicotinic acid hydrazide [isoniazid]) therapy are both acceptable means of therapy. BCG vaccination may be easier because it requires only one injection; however, the ability to perform future tuberculin skin testing is lost.

295. The answer is D (4). *(CDC/MMWR, December 6, 1985.)* Current data indicate that most pediatric cases of HTLV-III/LAV and AIDS infections are acquired perinatally from infected women. Transmission may occur during pregnancy, during labor and delivery, or in the immediate postpartum period. AIDS has also been reported in children delivered of HTLV-III/LAV positive mothers who underwent cesarean section. Therefore, no apparent protection is offered by this mode of delivery. Cesarean section should be reserved for obstetrical indications only. The rate of perinatal transmission varies widely between studies, but it is probably high, as high as 65 percent in one study. However, the transmission of disease from an infected mother to her infant is not absolute, as evidenced by healthy HTLV-III/LAV negative infants delivered to HTLV-III/LAV positive mothers. Current recommendations are that infected mothers should be advised to postpone pregnancy until further studies are done and more definite information can be obtained. HTLV-III/LAV has been isolated from breast milk of infected mothers and for this reason these mothers should be advised against breastfeeding to avoid any postnatal transmission.

296. The answer is D (4). *(Burrow, ed 2. pp 481–487. Pritchard, ed 17. pp 618–621.)* Studies of the effect of pregnancy on the course of systemic lupus erythematosus (SLE) have been inconsistent in their findings. Some studies suggest a worsening of the disease, while others show remission or no effect at all. If a woman who is informed that her lupus might get worse during pregnancy still wants to have a child, she may be supported in her plans. Women should be advised to await a clinical remission of the disease before attempting pregnancy, since the course of SLE is more favorable when pregnancy occurs during such a remission. In most cases therapeutic abortion is not indicated, because the postpartum flare-up, especially in renal disease, may occur whether the pregnancy has been terminated by abortion or delivery. For some very sick patients, however, abortion may be lifesaving. Only in cases involving severe renal disease does lupus seem to decrease the fertility rate.

297. The answer is A (1, 2, 3). *(Sciarra, ed 51, vol 3, chap 52, pp 1–7.)* Inactivated or formalin-killed vaccines such as those for influenza, typhoid fever, tetanus, pertussis, diphtheria toxoid, rabies, poliomyelitis, cholera, plague, and Rocky Mountain spotted fever are probably not hazardous for either the mother or the fetus. Among the live viral vaccines, such as those for measles, mumps, and poliomyelitis, only the rubella vaccine may retain its teratogenic properties. There is a 5 to 10 percent risk of fetal infection when the vaccine is administered during the first trimester. However, no cases of congenital rubella syndrome have been reported in this group of patients. Of the commonly administered, attenuated live viral vaccines, only polio virus has the ability to spread from a vaccine to susceptible individuals in the immediate environment. Therefore, the risk of infection for the pregnant mother who has been exposed to children who have recently been vaccinated for measles, mumps, and rubella is probably minimal.

298. The answer is B (1, 3). *(Burrow, ed 2. pp 202–209.)* Hyperthyroidism in pregnancy may cause neonatal thyrotoxicosis. The mechanism is not the transmission of triiodothyronine or thyroxine to the baby, but rather the crossing of long-acting thyroid stimulator (LATS) to the baby with subsequent hyperfunction of the fetal thyroid gland. Not all hyperthyroid women have LATS; and it is only those who do who are at risk for neonatal thyrotoxicosis. The usual treatment for hyperthyroidism in pregnancy is administration of thiourea compounds, although in some centers surgery is popular. Hyperthyroidism often becomes less severe during pregnancy, especially during the last trimester, at which time requirements for thiourea drugs often decrease. Because hyperthyroidism is a treatable disorder, it is not an indication for terminating a pregnancy.

299. The answer is E (all). *(Pritchard, ed 17. p 600.)* Maternal diabetes mellitus can affect a pregnant woman and her fetus in many ways. The development of preeclampsia or eclampsia is about four times as likely as among nondiabetic women. Infection also is more likely not only to occur but also to be severe. The incidences of fetal macrosomia or death and of dystocia are increased; and hydramnios is common. The likelihood of postpartum hemorrhage after vaginal delivery and the frequency of cesarean section both are increased in diabetic women.

300. The answer is A (1, 2, 3). *(Pritchard, ed 17. pp 779–780.)* Erythroblastosis fetalis, also known as isoimmune hemolytic disease of the newborn, results from the transplacental passage of maternal blood-group antibodies and subsequent destructive reaction with fetal erythrocyte antigens. It is theoretically possible for any blood-group antigen with the exceptions of Lewis and I antigens to cause erythroblastosis fetalis. Lewis and I antigens are not present on fetal red blood cells; furthermore, the antibodies to these two antigens are immunoglobulin M, which does not cross the placenta.

301. The answer is D (4). *(Burrow, ed 2. p 160.)* Eisenmenger's syndrome consists of severe pulmonary hypertension combined with a bidirectional or reversed shunt through a patent ductus arteriosus or an atrial or ventricular septal defect. The death rate during pregnancy for women who have this syndrome is higher than in any other form of congenital heart disease. Death usually occurs at or just after delivery and is probably associated with a sudden drop in peripheral vascular resistance. Atrial and ventricular septal defects, in the absence of pulmonary hypertension and right-to-left shunting, rarely cause problems during pregnancy. Unless shunting is minimal, a patent ductus arteriosus is usually detected by the time a woman becomes pregnant. Again, only reversal of the shunt should pose any problems.

302. The answer is D (4). *(Burrow, ed 2. pp 45–46.)* Although during early pregnancy the diabetogenic effects of placental hormones are not marked, there is still a net transfer of glucose from mother to fetus. For this reason, there is a tendency toward maternal hypoglycemia rather than hyperglycemia; ketoacidosis is rare and insulin reactions are common. In fact, one of the first symptoms of pregnancy in a diabetic woman may be hypoglycemia and decreasing insulin need. Later on in pregnancy, however, insulin requirements increase markedly and are about two-thirds higher than before pregnancy. Hypoglycemia then becomes less of a problem than ketoacidosis.

303. The answer is A (1, 2, 3). *(Burrow, ed 2. pp 195–199.)* It is not known why hypothyroidism is uncommon during pregnancy; however, the most widely supported explanation is that many hypothyroid patients are anovulatory and thus do not easily become pregnant. However, if a hypothyroid patient does become pregnant, her disease, if untreated, could lead to abortion and stillbirth. For this reason, most perinatologists prefer to treat hypothyroidism vigorously during pregnancy. For example, if a woman who has been placed on low-dose thyroid replacement for poorly documented hypothyroidism becomes pregnant, administration of thyroid hormone probably should be increased to full replacement dosage for the remainder of the pregnancy; after delivery, hormone therapy should be discontinued in order to reevaluate thyroid function.

304. The answer is C (2, 4). *(DiSaia, ed 2. pp 439–443.)* Ovarian neoplasms associated with pregnancy are usually benign; only 3 to 6 percent are found to be malignant. The neoplasms are most often unilateral when malignant. It has been estimated that 10 percent of ovarian masses discovered during pregnancy represent an enlarged, cystic corpus luteum. Transplacental spread of ovarian carcinoma to the fetus has not been documented.

305. The answer is B (1, 3). *(Pritchard, ed 17. pp 395–407.)* The patient described in the question presents with a classic history for abruption—that is, the sudden onset of abdominal pain accompanied by bleeding. Physical examination reveals a firm, tender uterus with frequent contractions, which confirms the diagnosis. The fact that a clot forms within 4 minutes suggests that coagulopathy is not present. Because abruption is often accompanied by hemorrhaging, it is important that appropriate fluids (i.e., lactated Ringer's solution and whole blood) be administered immediately to stabilize the mother's circulation. Cesarean section may be necessary in the case of a severe abruption, but only when fetal distress is evident or delivery is unlikely to be accomplished vaginally. Internal monitoring equipment should provide an early warning that the fetus is compromised. The internal uterine catheter provides pressure recordings, which are important if oxytocin stimulation is necessary. Generally, however, patients with abruptio placentae are contracting vigorously and do not need oxytocin.

306. The answer is B (1, 3). *(Burrow, ed 2. pp 13–16.)* Worldwide, the incidence of pregnancy-induced hypertension varies from a low of 2 percent in the Far East to almost 30 percent in Puerto Rico. Peak incidences occur in two groups: young primiparous women and multiparous women who are older than 35 years of age. Moreover, women who have had hypertension of pregnancy in the past have a 33 percent chance of developing the disease again in later pregnancies. Because of the difficulty in defining normal blood pressures for pregnant women, elevations in the systolic component of 20 mmHg or more or the diastolic component of 10 mmHg or more during pregnancy are defined as abnormal, notwithstanding the absolute blood pressure values. The terminology regarding hypertension in pregnancy is still in flux. The most inclusive term is hypertensive states of pregnancy. This is recommended by the American College of Obstetrics and Gynecology Committee on Terminology for general use. If the hypertension was not present before conception, then the term pregnancy-induced hypertension is also acceptable, but the term toxemia has fallen into disfavor.

307. The answer is E (all). *(Pritchard, ed 17. pp 395–407.)* Premature separation of the placenta (abruptio placentae) occurs in approximately 1 percent of all deliveries. Previous abruptio placentae, chronic hypertension, and pregnancy-induced hypertension all predispose to premature separation of the placenta. The placenta also is more likely than normal to separate between the birth of a first and second twin. Clinically, the severity of abruption ranges from a minimal amount of vaginal bleeding and rapid labor to massive hemorrhage, shock, consumptive coagulopathy, and fetal death. Clinical signs of abruption include an irritable, tender uterus, an enlarging uterus, hypertonic labor, and abdominal pain. Vaginal bleeding may or may not be present; in fact, some of the most severe abruptions with coagulopathies occur with "concealed hemorrhage," in which the retroplacental clot is contained within the uterus and has no egress to the vagina.

308. The answer is C (2, 4). *(Burrow, ed 2. pp 259–260.)* Hyperemesis gravidarum is intractable vomiting of pregnancy and is associated with disturbed nutrition. Early signs of the disorder include weight loss (up to 5 percent of body weight) and ketonuria. Because vomiting causes potassium loss, electrocardiographic evidence of potassium depletion, such as inverted T waves and prolonged Q-T and P-R intervals, is usually a later finding. Jaundice also is a later finding and probably is due to fatty infiltration of the liver; occasionally acute hepatic necrosis occurs. Hypokalemic nephropathy with isosthenuria may occur late. Hypoproteinemia also may result, caused by poor diet as well as by albuminuria. Patients who have hyperemesis gravidarum are best treated (if the disease is early in its course) with parenteral fluids and electrolytes, sedation, rest, vitamins, and antiemetics if necessary. In some cases, isolation of the patient is necessary. Very slow reinstitution of oral feeding is permitted after dehydration and electrolyte disturbances are corrected. Therapeutic abortion may be necessary in rare instances; usually, however, the disease improves spontaneously as pregnancy progresses.

309. The answer is A (1, 2, 3). *(Pritchard, ed 17. pp 415–416.)* When an incompetent cervix is suspected, weekly cervical examinations beginning at 16 to 18 weeks gestation can reveal evidence of cervical dilatation or effacement in time to perform corrective surgery. The most commonly used techniques are the Shirodkar cervical suture (cerclage), in which the purse-string suture is buried under the vaginal mucosa and the bladder pushed back for higher placement of the stitch, and the McDonald cervical suture, a simple purse-string suture most widely used when the cervix is well effaced. Once the diagnosis has been made, a cerclage procedure may be performed prophylactically in subsequent pregnancies, prior to any change in the cervix. This is best done at 14 to 16 weeks, well past the time when spontaneous abortion is common. Because it is not until 16 to 18 weeks that the fetus begins to occupy the lower uterine segment, it would be unlikely that incompetent cervix would be the cause of recurrent pregnancy loss at 14 to 16 weeks.

310–312. The answers are: 310-B, 311-D, 312-A. *(Pritchard, ed 17. pp 441–442, 459, 712–715.)* A circumvallate placenta contains a grayish-white ring located a variable distance from the edge of the placenta. The membranes (amnion and chorion) are folded over at this ring and are not in contact with the substance of the placenta peripheral to the ring. The fetal vessels do not go beyond the ring. Placenta circumvallata is associated with an increased rate of prematurity; why the rate is increased is unknown.

A succenturiate placenta is characterized by an accessory lobe apart from the main body of the placenta. Fetal vessels usually course through the membranes between the main and accessory lobes and can be identified on inspection of the membranes. If the fetal vessels on their way between the lobes should pass over the cervix, vasa praevia occurs. This condition is potentially dangerous, because the membranes may rupture, in turn rupturing a fetal vessel and causing fetal hemorrhage. If a succenturiate lobe is left within the uterus after the main body of the placenta has been delivered, postpartum hemorrhage can result; therefore, the presence of an accessory lobe should be checked for by intrauterine exploration.

Placenta accreta is a condition in which the usual plane of cleavage (Nitabuch's layer) between the placenta and decidua is absent and the villi attach to the myometrium. It is more common in women who have uterine scars, such as in the patient described in the question, and who have undergone previous cesarean section. Complications of placenta accreta are in part iatrogenic. An overly vigorous attempt at manual removal may cause uterine inversion or perforation and severe bleeding. A hysterectomy may be necessary, although leaving the placenta in place and treating the patient with methotrexate may suffice. Severe complications are most common with the more severe forms of placenta accreta. These forms are known as placenta increta, if the villi grow into the muscle of the uterus, and placenta percreta, if the placenta grows through the myometrium.

313–316. The answers are: 313-C, 314-E, 315-A, 316-D. *(Monif, ed 2. pp 156–159, 213–215, 278–284, 492–495.)* Group A β-hemolytic streptococci can cause puerperal or postoperative pelvic infection. Outbreaks of puerperal fever are still reported on obstetrical services, though not at anywhere near the frequency of 50 years ago. When the disease does occur, a point source among the hospital personnel should be suspected.

Group B β-hemolytic streptococci, which also can cause puerperal fever, have recently been recognized as a major cause of severe neonatal infection. The organism can be isolated from the cervices of about 5 percent of all pregnant women; infection of the infant, which can result in sepsis, occurs as the infant passes through the vagina.

Toxoplasma gondii, a protozoan parasite, is transmitted by flies from cat feces to human food. Thus, humans can become infected by consuming infected meat that is inadequately cooked or by coming in direct contact with feces of an infected cat. Acute toxoplasmosis in a pregnant woman may cause a fulminant fetal infection; infected neonates may be born with microcephaly, intracranial calcification, or other symptoms.

An effective attenuated-virus vaccine is available for immunization against rubella. However, its use is contraindicated for pregnant women and commonly is associated with development of arthralgia in adults.

317–321. The answers are: 317-D, 318-C, 319-C, 320-B, 321-E. *(Pritchard, ed 17. pp 395–411, 424–425, 467–473.)* Placenta previa is characterized by defective vascularization of the decidua, secondary to either inflammatory or atrophic changes; in this uncommon condition, the placenta is implanted over or near the internal os. Abruptio placentae (placenta abruption), which is associated very closely with maternal hypertension, is the premature separation of the placenta from the uterus. The Arias-Stella phenomenon, which refers to certain changes of the glands and epithelium of the endometrium, frequently is associated with ectopic pregnancy; however, this phenomenon also can occur whenever a conceptus is blighted and may be seen in intrauterine as well as extrauterine pregnancies. Spontaneous abortions histologically are accompanied by distended placental villi, hemorrhage into the decidua basalis, and evidence of necrotic changes in the region surrounding the hemorrhage.

Diagnosis and Management of Disorders of Labor, Delivery, and Puerperium

DIRECTIONS: Each question below contains five suggested responses. Select the **one best** response to each question.

322. Cesarean section confers an advantage to the survival of an infant in breech presentation in all the following situations EXCEPT

(A) a frank breech weighing 1000 to 1500 g
(B) a frank breech weighing 1500 to 4000 g
(C) an estimated fetal weight greater than 4000 g
(D) the presence of uterine dystocia
(E) a footling breech at term

323. A 30-year-old woman, para 6, is delivered vaginally following a precipitous labor with spontaneous delivery of an intact placenta. Excessive bleeding continues, despite manual exploration, bimanual massage, intravenous oxytocin, and administration of 0.2 mg Methergine IM. Which of the following is the next step in the management of this patient?

(A) Packing the uterus
(B) Immediate hysterectomy
(C) Bilateral hypogastric artery ligation
(D) IM injection of prostaglandin-$F_2\alpha$
(E) IV injection of 5 U oxytocin

Questions 324–325

A woman develops endometritis after a cesarean section has been performed. She is treated with penicillin and gentamicin but fails to respond.

324. Which of the following bacteria is resistant to these antibiotics and is likely to be responsible for this woman's infection?

(A) *Proteus mirabilis*
(B) *Bacteroides fragilis*
(C) *Escherichia coli*
(D) Alpha streptococci
(E) Anaerobic streptococci

325. The treatment of choice for this woman's condition would be

(A) polymyxin
(B) ampicillin
(C) cephalothin
(D) vancomycin
(E) clindamycin

326. The fetal monitoring strip shown below demonstrates which of the following?

(A) A uteroplacental insufficiency pattern
(B) A cord pattern
(C) Head compression
(D) Uneventful labor
(E) Fetal death

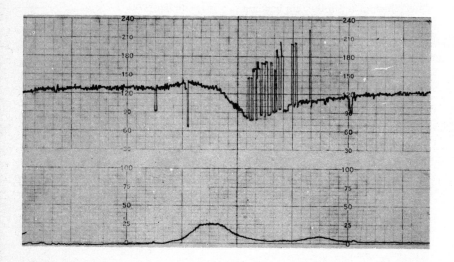

327. Which of the following abnormal presentations is an absolute indication for a vertical cesarean section incision?

(A) Single footling breech at term
(B) Double footling breech at term
(C) Complete breech at 32 weeks
(D) Back up transverse lie
(E) Back down transverse lie

Questions 328–329

A 24-year-old primigravid woman, who is intent on breast-feeding, decides upon a home delivery. Immediately after the birth of a 4.1-kg (9-lb) infant, the patient bleeds massively from extensive vaginal and cervical lacerations. She is brought in shock to the nearest hospital. Over 2 hours, 9 units of blood are transfused, and the blood pressure returns to a reasonable level. A hemoglobin value the next day is 7.5 g/100 ml, and 3 units of packed red blood cells are given.

328. The most likely late sequela to consider in this woman would be

(A) hemochromatosis
(B) Stein-Leventhal syndrome
(C) Sheehan syndrome
(D) Simmonds syndrome
(E) Cushing syndrome

329. Development of the sequela could be evident as early as

(A) 6 hours post partum
(B) 1 week post partum
(C) 1 month post partum
(D) 6 months post partum
(E) 1 year post partum

330. The graph below depicts a labor curve for a woman, gravida 2, para 1, with intact membranes. This labor curve is compatible with which of the following conditions?

(A) Normal labor
(B) Protracted latent phase
(C) Protracted active phase
(D) Primary dysfunction
(E) Hypertonic dysfunction

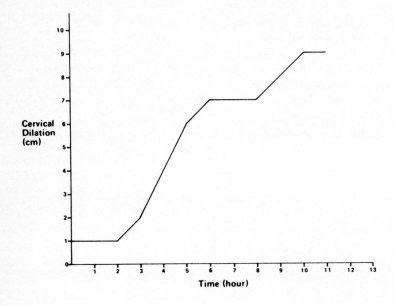

331. Important techniques to prevent aspiration pneumonitis following obstetrical general anesthesia include all the following EXCEPT

(A) fasting during labor
(B) antacid medications prior to anesthesia
(C) endotracheal intubation
(D) extubation with the patient in the lateral recumbent position with her head lowered
(E) extubation with the patient in the semierect position (semi-Fowler's)

332. Late deceleration patterns (type II dips) on a fetal monitoring strip represent

(A) cord compression
(B) pulmonary immaturity
(C) fetal hypoxia secondary to decreased perfusion of the intervillous spaces
(D) congenital cardiac conduction defects
(E) entry of the fetal head into the pelvic brim

333. Which of the following is the most appropriate management of a face presentation with no fetal distress and an adequate pelvis, as determined by digital examination?

(A) Perform immediate cesarean section without labor
(B) Allow spontaneous labor with vaginal delivery
(C) Perform forceps rotation in the second stage of labor to convert mentum posterior to mentum anterior and to allow vaginal delivery
(D) Allow to labor spontaneously until complete cervical dilatation is achieved, and then perform an internal podalic version with breech extraction
(E) Attempt manual conversion of the face to vertex in the second stage of labor

334. All the following statements about external cephalic version are true EXCEPT

(A) the use of general anesthesia is unacceptable in external versions
(B) amniotic fluid volume is a factor in determining whether a version should be performed
(C) prophylaxis prior to version with antiglobulin-D is recommended in Rh-negative mothers
(D) engagement of the presenting part is not considered a contraindication to version
(E) tocolysis with intravenous ritodrine has been shown to improve the results of external version

335. All the following are prerequi-
sites for the application of forceps EX-
CEPT

(A) engagement of the fetal vertex
(B) mentum anterior face presentation
(C) precise knowledge of the position
   of the vertex
(D) rupture of the membranes
(E) no evidence of fetal distress

DIRECTIONS: Each question below contains four suggested responses of which **one or more** is correct. Select

A	if	**1, 2, and 3**	are correct
B	if	**1 and 3**	are correct
C	if	**2 and 4**	are correct
D	if	**4**	is correct
E	if	**1, 2, 3, and 4**	are correct

336. Advantages of a lower segment transverse uterine incision over a lower segment vertical incision include

(1) less blood loss
(2) ease of repair
(3) less likelihood of adhesion to bowel or omentum along the incision line
(4) less likelihood of tearing into the uterine artery

337. Following a vaginal delivery, a woman develops a fever, lower abdominal pain, and uterine tenderness. She is alert, and her blood pressure and urine output are good. Large grampositive rods suggestive of *Clostridia* are seen in a smear of the cervix. Management should include

(1) close observation for renal failure or hemolysis
(2) immediate radiographic examination for gas in the uterus
(3) high-dose antibiotic therapy
(4) hysterectomy

338. Barton forceps can be described by which of the following statements?

(1) It is useful when the fetal head is in a transverse position in a platypelloid pelvis
(2) It is useful when traction and rotation are to be performed simultaneously
(3) Application of the blades can be adjusted by a sliding lock
(4) The posterior blade is hinged

339. Hypertonic dysfunctional labor generally can be expected to

(1) cause little pain
(2) occur in the active phase of labor
(3) react favorably to oxytocin stimulation
(4) respond to sedation

340. A 25-year-old woman has recently delivered a 4-kg (8½-lb) boy and is now experiencing heavy vaginal bleeding. The obstetrician should rule out which of the following causes of postpartum hemorrhage?

(1) Uterine atony
(2) Vaginal/cervical lacerations
(3) Retained placental fragments
(4) Blood dyscrasias

		SUMMARY OF DIRECTIONS		
A	**B**	**C**	**D**	**E**
1,2,3 only	1,3 only	2,4 only	4 only	All are correct

341. Fetal presenting positions that are usually undeliverable vaginally include

(1) brow
(2) mentum anterior
(3) mentum posterior
(4) left sacrum posterior

342. Chorioamnionitis develops in a woman whose membranes have ruptured at 35 weeks gestation; the fetus is alive. Management should include

(1) systemic antibiotics
(2) high-dose corticosteroids
(3) delivery by either a brief induction or cesarean section
(4) heparinization

343. A genital tract infection after delivery (puerperal infection) is characterized by which of the following statements?

(1) A temperature of 38°C (100.4°F) or higher on any 2 of the first 10 postpartum days (excluding the first day) is considered the standard definition of puerperal morbidity
(2) Iatrogenic causes are significant sources of infection
(3) The most common pathogens involved are those that normally inhabit the bowel and lower genital tract
(4) Anaerobic infections are common and frequently are caused by *Bacteroides, Peptostreptococcus,* or *Clostridium*

DIRECTIONS: Each group of questions below consists of lettered headings followed by a set of numbered items. For each numbered item select the **one** lettered heading with which it is **most** closely associated. Each lettered heading may be used **once, more than once, or not at all.**

Questions 344–347

For each clinical situation described below, choose the appropriate type of obstetrical forceps.

    (A) Simpson forceps
    (B) Kielland forceps
    (C) Barton forceps
    (D) Chamberlen forceps
    (E) Piper forceps

344. A breech delivery with an aftercoming head

345. The occiput transverse position in a flat pelvis

346. Fetal rotation

347. An elective low forceps delivery

Questions 348–350

For each of the following clinical descriptions, select the procedure that would be most appropriate.

    (A) External version
    (B) Internal version
    (C) Midforceps rotation
    (D) Low transverse cesarean section
    (E) Classic cesarean section

348. A 24-year-old primigravid woman, at term, has been in labor for 16 hours and has been dilated to 9 cm for 3 hours. The fetal vertex is in the right occiput posterior position, at +1 station, and molded. There have been mild late decelerations for the last 30 minutes. Twenty minutes ago, the fetal scalp pH was 7.27; it is now 7.20

349. A 24-year-old woman (gravida 3, para 2) is at 40 weeks gestation. The fetus is in the transverse lie presentation

350. You have just delivered an infant weighing 2.5 kg (5.5 lb) at 39 weeks gestation. Because the uterus still feels large, you do a vaginal examination. A second set of membranes is bulging through a fully dilated cervix, and you feel a small part presenting in the sac. A fetal heart is auscultated at 60 beats per minute

Diagnosis and Management of Disorders of Labor, Delivery, and Puerperium

Answers

322. The answer is B. *(Pritchard, ed 17. pp 651–659.)* At any time in pregnancy, the breech presentation yields a higher perinatal morbidity, but perinatal mortality for the frank breech at term is the same regardless of the mode of delivery.

Perinatal mortality of the breech presentation can be reduced by the use of a cesarean section in any type of breech presentation between 1000 and 1500 g or over 4000 g. Mortality is also lower if a cesarean section is used to deliver any breech presentation other than a frank breech, regardless of the fetal weight. It has been observed that higher mortality and lower Apgar scores are seen in breech labor requiring augmentation.

323. The answer is D. *(Pritchard, ed 17. pp 707–712.)* The management of severe third-stage bleeding involves stabilization of the patient with fluid and blood replacement; examination of the cervix and vagina for lacerations; and exploration of the uterine cavity for retained placental fragments, accessory lobes, and uterine rupture. Once uterine atony is determined as the cause of excessive bleeding, immediate treatment involves IV oxytocin as a dilute solution, while massaging the uterus bimanually. Methergine intramuscularly is used in cases of oxytocin failure. Prostaglandin-$F_2\alpha$ has been proved successful in preventing postpartum hemorrhage caused by uterine atony, and it should be administered prior to performing surgery. There is no therapeutic advantage of a uterine pack in preventing postpartum hemorrhage.

324. The answer is B. *(Monif, ed 2. pp 8, 169–172.)* Infections caused by *Bacteroides fragilis*, a gram-negative anaerobic bacillus, are a significant obstetrical problem. Not only is the organism resistant to many commonly used antibiotics (including penicillin and gentamicin), but it is difficult to isolate, culture, and identify as well. The high incidence of gynecological and obstetrical *B. fragilis* infections may be due to the pathogen's predominance among the anaerobic bacteria of the lower bowel. Although the other organisms listed in the question also can cause postpartum infection, they are sensitive to antibiotic therapy with penicillin and gentamicin.

325. The answer is E. *(Monif, ed 2. pp 8, 172–176.)* Clindamycin is the most effective antibiotic for treating women who have bacteroidosis. Chloramphenicol and tetracycline are alternative choices for antibiotic therapy in nonpregnant women; however, tetracycline-resistant strains of *B. fragilis* may be emerging. Lincomycin and erythromycin also can be effective in the management of affected women.

326. The answer is A. *(Lin, pp 319–327.)* The fetal monitoring strip that accompanies the question illustrates a uteroplacental insufficiency pattern. In this pattern, deceleration of the heart rate begins after the onset of the contraction, and the lowest rate occurs after the contraction has peaked. In addition there is a very slow return to the baseline. This is an ominous pattern and implies significant fetal hypoxia. Scalp pH sampling is warranted in this situation; and if acidosis is present and the pattern persists with subsequent contractions, rapid delivery should be performed. Diabetes mellitus and hypertensive states of pregnancy are diseases that typically compromise the functional capacity of the placenta.

327. The answer is E. *(Pritchard, ed 17. pp 665–666.)* All the listed abnormal presentations may, under various circumstances, be approached best via a vertical uterine incision. The back down transverse lie, however, requires a vertical incision since it allows neither the vertex nor the feet to gain proximity to a lower uterine transverse incision.

328–329. The answers are: 328-C, 329-B. *(Pritchard, ed 17. pp 707–709.)* A disadvantage of home delivery is the lack of facilities to control postpartum hemorrhage. The woman described in the question delivered a large baby, suffered multiple soft-tissue injuries, and went into shock, needing 9 units of blood by the time she reached the hospital. Sheehan syndrome seems a likely possibility in this woman. This syndrome of anterior pituitary necrosis related to obstetrical hemorrhage can be diagnosed by 1 week post partum, as lactation fails to commence normally. Although many modern women choose hormonal therapy to prevent lactation, the woman described in the question was intent on breast-feeding and so would not have received suppressant. She therefore could have been expected to begin lactation at the usual time. Other symptoms of Sheehan syndrome include amenorrhea, atrophy of the breasts, and loss of thyroid and adrenal function.

The other presented choices for late sequelae are rather far-fetched. Hemochromatosis would not be expected to occur in this healthy young woman, especially since she did not receive prolonged transfusions. Cushing, Simmonds, and Stein-Leventhal syndromes are not known to be related to postpartum hemorrhage.

It is important to note that home delivery is not a predisposing factor to postpartum hemorrhage.

330. The answer is C. *(Pritchard, ed 17. pp 314–315, 641–644.)* The labor depicted by the curve in the question is characteristic of a protracted active phase. That the woman has entered the active phase is evident by the rate of dilatation (from 2 cm to 7 cm) over the space of 3 hours. The normal active phase progresses at a rate of at least 1.5 cm/hour in a multiparous woman and 1.2 cm/hour in a nulliparous woman. After 7 cm dilatation is reached in this patient, however, progress slows down to 2 cm over the next 4 hours, or 0.5 cm/hour, and the active phase is said to be protracted. Another name for this condition is secondary arrest of labor. (Primary arrest of labor is arrest of progress before the active phase has begun.) If this woman's contractions are adequate by intrauterine monitoring and further progress does not occur, most obstetricians would perform a cesarean section. If hypotonic dysfunction were causing the protracted labor, some obstetricians would stimulate contractions with intravenous oxytocin.

331. The answer is E. *(Pritchard, ed 17. pp 356–358.)* Aspiration pneumonitis is the most common cause of anesthetic-related death in obstetrics. Its occurrence may be minimized by reducing both the volume and acidity of gastric contents, which is often difficult in the patient in labor whose stomach is extremely slow to empty. All obstetrical patients should be intubated for general anesthesia by a skilled individual. Extubation must be accomplished only after the patient is fully conscious and recumbent with her head turned to the side and lowered below the level of her chest.

332. The answer is C. *(Lin, p 319–327.)* Late deceleration patterns on a fetal monitoring strip result from fetal hypoxia caused by decreased perfusion, during contractions, of the intervillous spaces. A healthy fetus can tolerate the transient hypoxia resulting from contractions without exhibiting heart rate changes. Thus, late deceleration patterns are ominous, because they indicate that a fetus has very little reserve. Permanent damage of the central nervous system can result if the hypoxia is allowed to persist.

333. The answer is B. *(Pritchard, ed 17. p 660.)* In the presence of a face presentation, successful vaginal delivery will occur the majority of the time with an adequate pelvis. Spontaneous internal rotation during labor is required to bring the chin to the anterior position, which allows the neck to pass beneath the pubis. Therefore, the patient is allowed to labor spontaneously; a cesarean section is employed for failure to progress or for fetal distress. Manual conversion to vertex, forceps rotation, and internal version are no longer employed in obstetrics to deliver the face presentation because of undue trauma to both the mother and the fetus.

334. The answer is D. *(Pritchard, ed 17. pp 656–657, 864–866.)* The use of external cephalic version is gaining popularity as a safe alternative to term breech presentation, and it is recommended by many, but not all, obstetricians in uncomplicated pregnancies with a breech or a transverse lie after 36 weeks. The criteria for a safe and successful external version include continuous fetal heart rate monitoring, a nonirritable uterus, a sufficient quantity of amniotic fluid, and a presenting part that is not engaged in the pelvis. The availability of ultrasound and the capability of performing an emergency cesarean section are also strongly recommended. The use of tocolytics is advocated and has been shown to improve the success of version, especially on repeat versions after a previous failure. General anesthesia is contraindicated because of the likelihood of trauma to the mother and the fetus. Antiglobulin-D prophylaxis is recommended prior to external version in all Rh-negative women because of the risk of fetal-maternal bleeding with manipulation of the uterus.

335. The answer is E. *(Pritchard, ed 17. pp 840–841.)* Before forceps can be safely applied to the fetal vertex, certain conditions must be met. Descent of the vertex into the pelvis must have taken place. The presentation should be vertex or face, with the mentum anterior; and the cervix must be completely dilated. The membranes must be ruptured, and the precise position of the vertex within the pelvis must be known prior to application of the forceps. Finally, forceps should not be applied if there is obvious disproportion of the fetal vertex to any plane of the bony pelvis. The presence or absence of fetal distress is not a prerequisite for the application of forceps.

336. The answer is A (1, 2, 3). *(Pritchard, ed 17. p 871.)* The lower segment transverse uterine incision (curve technique) offers many advantages over the vertical uterine incision. Less blood loss, ease of repair, less omental and bowel adhesion, less likelihood of tearing into the cervix and vagina, and less likelihood of rupturing along the incision line in future pregnancies are all advantages of the transverse uterine incision. The vertical incision is less likely to tear into the uterine vessels, and it does offer the advantage of more room, if necessary, for the abnormal lie of the fetus.

337. The answer is A (1, 2, 3). *(Monif, ed 2. pp 178–188.)* *Clostridia* can be seen in 5 to 10 percent of pelvic cultures. When the organism is found, appropriate antibiotic therapy (e.g., with penicillin) and close observation for gas gangrene, hemolysis, and renal failure are in order. Presumed identification on the basis of Gram stain alone or the presence of a mild infection without signs of sepsis or extrauterine involvement is not reason enough to proceed to hysterectomy.

338. The answer is B (1, 3). *(Pritchard, ed 17. p 846.)* A special feature of Barton forceps is the hinged anterior blade. This type of forceps is useful when the fetal head is in a transverse position in a platypelloid pelvis; it should not be used, however, to perform simultaneous traction and rotation. Application of the forceps is by moving the hinged blade about the occiput or face; adjustment is made by a sliding lock.

339. The answer is D (4). *(Pritchard, ed 17. p 647.)* Hypertonic uterine dysfunction is characterized by a lack of coordination of uterine contractions, possibly caused by disorganization of the contraction gradient, which normally is greatest at the fundus and least at the cervix. This type of dysfunction usually appears during the latent phase of labor and is responsive to sedation, not oxytocin stimulation. The disorder is accompanied by a great deal of discomfort with little cervical dilatation (the familiar and painful false labor). After being sedated for a few hours, affected women usually awaken in active labor.

340. The answer is E (all). *(Pritchard, ed 17. pp 707–708.)* Undoubtedly the most common cause of postpartum hemorrhage in the early puerperium is uterine atony, but vaginal lacerations and retained placental fragments must also be considered. Once these three major causes of hemorrhage have been ruled out, disorders of the coagulation system, either congenital (e.g., von Willebrand's disease) or acquired (e.g., disseminated intravascular coagulation), should be considered. The initial assessment of the woman described in the question should include a determination of previous bleeding problems, time since delivery, special problems encountered during delivery (e.g., manual removal of the placenta or vaginal laceration), quantity of blood loss, vital signs (including positional effect on blood pressure), and uterine consistency. Further diagnostic or therapeutic steps would depend upon this initial assessment of causative factors.

341. The answer is B (1, 3). *(Pritchard, ed 17. pp 660–662.)* In brow presentation, the fetal head is midway between flexion and extension. Except with an extremely small baby, engagement cannot occur unless flexion to vertex or extension to face presentation supervenes. In face presentation, delivery is by flexion rather than extension as in vertex presentations. Only the mentum anterior is capable of flexing under the pubic symphysis. The mentum posterior position does not allow flexion, because the neck is too short to go around the sacrum. The left sacrum posterior position is a variation of breech presentation. Although many present-day obstetricians would rarely deliver a breech vaginally, the breech presentation is by no means undeliverable.

342. The answer is B (1, 3). *(Monif, ed 2. pp 369–370.)* The main mode of treatment for women who have chorioamnionitis is delivery. If the cervix is effaced and dilated, a brief induction could be undertaken; if the cervix is unripe, then abdominal delivery would be in order. Administration of potent antibiotics is important to prevent the development of sepsis in the mother. Although corticosteroids are not indicated in the treatment of women who have uncomplicated chorioamnionitis, such therapy might be valuable if septic shock develops. The use of steroids to accelerate pulmonary maturity would be inappropriate. Heparinization is not indicated in uncomplicated chorioamnionitis. Coagulation disorders, which may be a complication of severe infection, should not be treated unless there is uncontrollable bleeding.

343. The answer is E (all). *(Pritchard, ed 17. pp 719–729.)* The agents most responsible for puerperal infections are those normally found in the lower genital tract or in the bowel. These agents may be anaerobic bacteria (most commonly *Bacteroides, Peptostreptococcus,* and *Clostridium*) or aerobic bacteria (such as *Escherichia coli, Klebsiella, Pseudomonas,* and *Enterobacter*); infections caused by a combination of two or more pathogens occur frequently. Most puerperal infections are wound infections; trauma before or during delivery and iatrogenic bacterial contamination are significant etiological factors. Puerperal morbidity is defined as a temperature of 38°C (100.4°F) or higher occurring on any 2 of the first 10 postpartum days, excluding the first.

344–347. The answers are: 344-E, 345-C, 346-B, 347-A. *(Pritchard, ed 17. pp 837–853, 859–864.)* Piper forceps were designed specifically for the delivery of the after-coming head in a vaginal breech delivery. They should never be applied until the head has fully entered the maternal pelvis and is engaged.

Barton forceps are designed for a transverse arrest in a platypelloid (flat) pelvis. The pelvic curve of the forceps is in an appropriate position via-à-vis the maternal pelvis when the forceps are applied to the occiput transverse. Descent is then accomplished in this position, and rotation to the occiput anterior does not occur until the pelvic floor is reached. Rotation in the midplane thus is unnecessary; indeed, such rotation would be difficult in a flat pelvis.

Kielland forceps are designed specifically for rotation. They have very little pelvic curve and thus are unlikely to cause maternal soft-tissue injury during rotation. They can be used for occiput posterior or transverse positions, in which rotation is planned before traction is applied.

Simpson forceps are the prototype forceps for the molded head. They are useful for low forceps deliveries, and some obstetricians use Simpson or similar forceps for various rotation maneuvers.

Chamberlen forceps, the first true obstetrical forceps, were in use in the late sixteenth century.

348–350. The answers are: 348-D, 349-A, 350-B. *(Pritchard, ed 17. pp 520, 662–666, 840, 867–868, 878–879. Romney, ed 2. p 669.)* A woman who has been dilated 9 cm for 3 hours is experiencing a secondary arrest in labor. The deteriorating fetal condition (as evidenced, for example, by late decelerations and falling scalp pH) dictates immediate delivery. A forceps rotation would be inappropriate because the cervix is not fully dilated. Cesarean section would be the safest and most expeditious method. Classic cesarean section is rarely used now because of greater blood loss and a higher incidence in subsequent pregnancies of rupture of the scar prior to labor. The best procedure would be a low transverse cesarean section.

A transverse lie is undeliverable vaginally. One treatment option is to do nothing and hope that the lie will be longitudinal by the time labor commences. The only other appropriate maneuver would be to perform an external cephalic version. This maneuver should be done in the hospital, with monitoring of the fetal heart. If the version is successful and the cervix is ripe, it might be best to take advantage of the favorable vertex position by rupturing the membranes at that point and inducing labor.

According to some studies, 25 percent of twins are diagnosed at the time of delivery. Although sonography or radiography can diagnose multiple gestation early in pregnancy, these methods are not used routinely in all medical centers. The second twin is probably the only remaining situation where internal version is permissible. Although some obstetricians might perform a cesarean section for a second twin presenting as a footling or shoulder, fetal bradycardia dictates that immediate delivery be done; and internal podalic version is the quickest procedure.

CLINICAL
GYNECOLOGY

Menstrual and Endocrine Disorders

DIRECTIONS: Each question below contains five suggested responses. Select the **one best** response to each question.

351. All the following are associated with hyperprolactinemia/amenorrhea EXCEPT

(A) hypoestrogenism
(B) hypothyroidism
(C) pituitary adenoma
(D) anorexia nervosa
(E) galactorrhea

352. The presence of a uterus and fallopian tubes in an otherwise phenotypically normal male is due to

(A) lack of müllerian inhibiting factor
(B) lack of testosterone
(C) increased levels of estrogens
(D) 46,XX karyotype
(E) presence of ovarian tissue early in embryonic development

353. A 35-year-old woman presents with hypotension, cold intolerance, amenorrhea, waxy skin with multiple fine wrinkles, loss of axillary and pubic hair, and loss of skin pigmentation. Her urine sodium levels are normal. The most likely diagnosis is

(A) hypothyroidism
(B) Addison's disease
(C) panhypopituitarism
(D) malignant melanoma
(E) diabetes insipidus

354. In a 29-year-old woman taking oral contraceptives, amenorrhea is most likely due to

(A) pregnancy
(B) pituitary tumor
(C) Asherman's syndrome
(D) relative progesterone excess in the contraceptive
(E) relative estrogen excess in the contraceptive

355. Androgens are predominantly produced in the adrenal gland or ovary. The most clinically useful hormonal measurement to differentiate between ovarian and adrenal production is

(A) testosterone/free testosterone
(B) dehydroepiandrosterone sulfate (DHAS)
(C) dehydroepiandrosterone
(D) dehydrotestosterone (DHT)
(E) androstenedione

DIRECTIONS: Each question below contains four suggested responses of which **one or more** is correct. Select

A	if	**1, 2, and 3**	are correct
B	if	**1 and 3**	are correct
C	if	**2 and 4**	are correct
D	if	**4**	is correct
E	if	**1, 2, 3, and 4**	are correct

356. Causes of precocious puberty in girls include

(1) estrogen-producing ovarian tumors
(2) head trauma
(3) polyostotic fibrous dysplasia (Albright syndrome)
(4) hypothyroidism

357. Increased incidences of endometrial hyperplasia and endometrial carcinoma have been described in patients with which of the following?

(1) Infertility
(2) Theca cell tumors of the ovary
(3) Polycystic ovaries
(4) Ingestion of conjugated estrogens

358. True statements regarding the empty-sella syndrome include which of the following?

(1) Headache is a common complaint
(2) Most affected patients have visual field defects
(3) It is most commonly seen in middle-aged, obese women
(4) X-ray of the sella turcica often reveals asymmetrical enlargement

359. A pubertal response to luteinizing hormone releasing hormone (LRH) or a prominent increase in the luteinizing hormone (LH) pulses during sleep would be seen in patients with

(1) iatrogenic sexual precocity
(2) premature thelarche
(3) granulosa cell tumors
(4) idiopathic/constitutional precocious puberty

360. Areas of the body that develop hair in response to sexual hormones include the

(1) face
(2) pubic area
(3) chest
(4) lower abdomen

361. A 19-year-old woman consults you because of amenorrhea and galactorrhea of 1 year's duration. Her periods previously had been regular. She has had no other symptoms except for a mild headache. Diagnoses compatible with the findings on the CAT scan shown below include

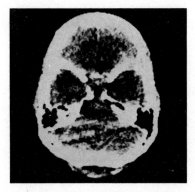

(1) empty-sella syndrome
(2) amenorrhea of a nonpituitary etiology
(3) microadenoma of the pituitary gland
(4) suprasellar lesion of a pituitary adenoma

362. Mammary-gland development is a common feature of patients who have

(1) testicular feminization
(2) Reifenstein syndrome
(3) Klinefelter syndrome
(4) Turner syndrome

363. Amenorrhea-galactorrhea is associated with

(1) hypothyroidism
(2) discontinuation of oral contraceptives
(3) abnormalities of the sella turcica
(4) the puerperium

364. A 19-year-old patient presents to your office with primary amenorrhea. She has normal breast development, but the uterus is absent. Diagnostic possibilities include

(1) testicular feminization
(2) gonadal dysgenesis
(3) müllerian agenesis
(4) Klinefelter syndrome

365. True statements concerning anorexia nervosa include which of the following?

(1) It is seen predominantly in females, rarely in males
(2) Most affected patients have an obsessive-compulsive personality
(3) Mean 24-hour concentration of cortisol is twice normal
(4) Thyroid hormones are in the normal range

366. In a patient presenting with primary amenorrhea, who has normal breast and reproductive organ development, the initial workup should include which of the following studies?

(1) Prolactin
(2) FSH-LH
(3) TSH
(4) Karyotype

367. Asherman syndrome is characterized by which of the following?

(1) Biphasic basal body temperatures
(2) Diagnosis by endometrial biopsy
(3) Amenorrhea
(4) Remission after removal of an intrauterine device

SUMMARY OF DIRECTIONS

A	B	C	D	E
1,2,3 only	1,3 only	2,4 only	4 only	All are correct

368. The causes of panhypopituitarism include

(1) postpartum hemorrhage
(2) Hand-Schüller-Christian disease
(3) temporal arteritis
(4) empty-sella syndrome

369. Signs or symptoms commonly associated with anorexia nervosa but NOT with hypopituitarism include

(1) marked wasting
(2) loss of axillary and pubic hair
(3) elevated levels of human growth hormone
(4) decreased thyroid activity

370. Endometrial dysfunctional bleeding includes which of the following types?

(1) Estrogen breakthrough bleeding
(2) Estrogen withdrawal bleeding
(3) Progesterone breakthrough bleeding
(4) Progesterone withdrawal bleeding

371. Medications useful in the management of patients with hirsutism include

(1) danazol
(2) spironolactone
(3) phenytoin
(4) cimetidine

372. Suggested treatment modalities for premenstrual syndrome include

(1) progesterone
(2) spironolactone
(3) antiprostaglandins
(4) vitamin therapy

373. Medical therapy for primary dysmenorrhea includes

(1) prostaglandin inhibitors
(2) analgesics
(3) inhibitors of ovulation
(4) oxytocin

374. Delayed puberty and sexual infantilism, secondary to hypogonadotropic hypogonadism, can be seen in patients with

(1) renal disease
(2) hypothyroidism
(3) Cushing's disease
(4) anorexia nervosa

DIRECTIONS: Each group of questions below consists of lettered headings followed by a set of numbered items. For each numbered item select the **one** lettered heading with which it is **most** closely associated. Each lettered heading may be used **once, more than once, or not at all.**

Questions 375–379

For each description that follows, select the type of sexual precocity with which it is most likely to be associated.

(A) True sexual precocity
(B) Incomplete sexual precocity
(C) Isosexual precocious pseudo-puberty
(D) Heterosexual precocious pseudopuberty
(E) Precocity due to gonadotropin-producing tumors

375. Defined by the presence of virilizing signs in girls

376. Characterized by the presence of premature adrenarche, pubarche, or thelarche

377. Can arise from cranial tumors or hypothyroidism

378. Stems from premature activation of the hypothalamus-pituitary system

379. Frequently caused by ovarian tumors

Questions 380–383

For each patient described below, select the medication or testing suited to correct or diagnose the dysfunctional bleeding.

(A) Clomiphene citrate (Clomid)
(B) Oral contraceptives
(C) Antiprostaglandin
(D) Endometrial sampling
(E) None of the above

380. A 24-year-old sexually active woman presents with irregular cycles at intervals anywhere from 30 to 90 days. Menstrual flow is usually heavy, and she has noted increasing hirsutism

381. A 52-year-old, obese, hypertensive woman presents with abnormal bleeding

382. A 15-year-old girl, who is not sexually active, complains of excessively heavy menstrual flow with associated dysmenorrhea

383. A 32-year-old infertility patient with intermenstrual spotting had an endometrial biopsy that was interpreted as revealing an inadequate luteal phase

Menstrual and Endocrine Disorders
Answers

351. The answer is D. *(Speroff, ed 3. pp 163–179.)* Elevated levels of prolactin can be seen in patients with hypo- or hyperthyroidism, pituitary adenomas, galactorrhea, or chronic renal failure. A number of drugs have been associated with elevated prolactin including phenothiazines, metoclopramide, reserpine, and methyldopa. Approximately one third of patients with secondary amenorrhea will have a pituitary adenoma, and this incidence increases if galactorrhea is also present. The elevated prolactin appears to suppress the pulsatile secretion of gonadotropin releasing-hormone, and thus the patient becomes amenorrheal and hypoestrogenic, although not all patients with elevated prolactin will become amenorrheal. Hormonal changes in anorexia nervosa include elevated cortisol, low FSH/LH, normal prolactin, decreased T_3, high reverse T_3, and normal TSH.

352. The answer is A. *(Speroff, ed 3. p 353.)* Individuals who appear to be normal males but who possess a uterus and tubes have an isolated failure of müllerian inhibiting factor. Their karyotype is 46,XY, testes are present, and testosterone production is normal.

353. The answer is C. *(Wilson, ed 7. pp 188–189.)* The most likely diagnosis of the woman described in the question is panhypopituitarism. The associated hypotension results from a decrease in cortisone production, which is caused by a lack of corticotropin. Because the adrenal glands still maintain the ability to produce aldosterone, sodium levels are usually unchanged. Cold intolerance, amenorrhea, and changes in skin appearance and pigmentation are frequent signs of hypopituitarism. A patient who has hypothyroidism generally would present with different symptoms from those described, although cold intolerance may be encountered. A patient with Addison's disease would not be able to maintain body sodium. Malignant melanoma causes none of the presenting features described; and although diabetes insipidus may be a symptom of hypopituitarism, it does not cause the described symptomatology.

354. The answer is D. *(Speroff, ed 3. pp 436–437.)* In all birth-control pill combinations the progestational effect dominates and produces a relatively shallow, atrophic endometrium that may be inadequate to yield withdrawal bleeding in some patients. This is reversible with resumption of normal ovarian function or estrogen supplementation.

355. The answer is B. *(Speroff, ed 3. pp 205–211.)* Testosterone is produced both in the adrenal gland and the ovary with each contributing approximately 25 percent. Fifty percent of testosterone production is from the peripheral conversion of androstenedione. Androstenedione is produced in equal amounts by the adrenal gland and the ovary. Although 90 percent of the dehydroepiandrosterone is produced in the adrenal gland, the ovary contributes approximately 10 percent. Dehydroepiandrosterone sulfate (DHAS) is produced entirely by the adrenal gland. DHAS is elevated slightly in patients with polycystic ovarian disease. Significant elevations occur with adrenal tumors or adrenal hyperplasia. Differentiation is assessed by the patient's ability to suppress DHAS after dexamethazone therapy.

356. The answer is E (all). *(Speroff, ed 3. pp 370–376.)* The most common cause of true sexual precocious puberty is constitutional or idiopathic. Cerebral problems causing precocious development include tumors, infections, hydrocephaly, and trauma. Precocious puberty can also be seen in patients with hypothyroidism, polyostotic fibrous dysplasia, neurofibromatosis, and other disorders. True sexual precocity is characterized by elevated gonadotropin levels and a normal ovulatory pattern. It represents premature activation of a normally operating hypothalamus-pituitary relationship. Pseudoprecocious puberty is a situation in which the maturing normal gonads are not the source of the excess sexual steroids. This can be seen in patients with ovarian or adrenal tumors. Sexual development can either be isosexual, caused by estrogen production, or heterosexual, caused by androgen production. The most common ovarian tumor is the granulosa cell tumor.

357. The answer is E (all). *(Kase, pp 860–861.)* Much evidence supports the relationship of unopposed estrogen and anovulation to hyperplasia of the endometrium. Any condition that increases endogenous estrogen levels, especially without regular progesterone challenges, may predispose the patient to uterine cancer.

358. The answer is B (1, 3). *(Speroff, ed 3. p 170.)* The empty-sella syndrome is a well-known condition in which an extension of the subarachnoid space is formed by the sella turcica. Pneumoencephalography, which will fill this space with air, is used as a diagnostic tool. Sella turcica x-ray usually reveals symmetrical enlargements. Individuals affected by this syndrome are frequently middle-aged women who are obese. The symptoms are generally nonspecific, with headaches being the most common complaint. The empty-sella syndrome is a benign condition that does not lead to pituitary failure. Inadvertent treatment for a pituitary tumor is probably the greatest hazard to the patient.

359. The answer is D (4). *(Speroff, ed 3. pp 364–365.)* Normal signs of puberty involve breast budding (thelarche, 9.8 years), pubic hair (pubarche, 10.5 years), and menarche (12.8 years). Besides an increase in androgens and a moderate rise in FSH and LH levels, one of the first indications of puberty is an increase in the amplitude and frequency of nocturnal LH pulses. In patients with idiopathic true precocious puberty, the pituitary response to LRH is identical to that in girls undergoing normal puberty. Iatrogenic sexual precocity (i.e., the accidental ingestion of estrogens), premature thelarche, and ovarian tumors are examples of sexual precocity independent of LH function.

360. The answer is E (all). *(Speroff, ed 3. pp 205–211.)* Areas of the body with hair responding to sexual hormones include the face, lower abdomen, anterior thighs, chest, breast, axilla, and pubic area. One must also recognize that there are racial and ethnic variations in the number and thickness of hair follicles. Signs of androgen excess besides increased hair growth, in order of increasing serum hormone levels, are acne, oily skin, menstrual irregularity, increased libido, clitoromegaly, and frank masculinization.

361. The answer is A (1, 2, 3). *(Speroff, ed 3. pp 153–156.)* The CAT scan that accompanies the question depicts a coronal section of the skull; the midline spherical area represents the sella turcica. In this study, the sella turcica is perfectly symmetric and normal in size. In the empty-sella syndrome, the sella is basically normal in configuration; a portion of arachnoid membrane herniates down through the diaphragm and compresses the active pituitary gland. Because microadenomas of the pituitary gland, which can produce prolactin and thus cause amenorrhea and galactorrhea, are usually less than 5 mm in size, they would not appear in the CAT scan shown. A suprasellar lesion of the pituitary gland would be larger than 5 mm and therefore would appear on most CAT scans.

362. The answer is A (1, 2, 3). *(Wilson, ed 7. pp 178, 409, 1312.)* The degree of mammary-gland development depends on the relationship between estrogen and androgen production and utilization. Development of mammary tissue is significant in individuals who have testicular feminization, in which peripheral testosterone use is very low; Reifenstein syndrome, in which serum testosterone levels are reduced; or Klinefelter syndrome, in which testosterone production is decreased but estrogen production remains normal or near normal. On the other hand, mammary-gland development is not characteristic of patients with Turner syndrome, who produce no androgen and very little estrogen.

363. The answer is E (all). *(Speroff, ed 3. pp 251–254.)* Amenorrhea and galactorrhea may be seen with all the listed clinical states. The differential diagnosis is difficult because of the multiple possible causes. For example, excessive estrogens such as with birth-control pills can reduce prolactin inhibiting factor (PIF), as can intensive suckling. Phenothiazine-derivative drugs are also known to have mammotrophic properties. Hypothyroidism appears to cause galactorrhea secondary to thyrotropin releasing hormone (TRH) stimulation of prolactin. With persistent elevated prolactin levels without obvious cause (e.g., breast-feeding), an evaluation for pituitary adenoma becomes necessary.

364. The answer is B (1, 3). *(Speroff, ed 3. pp 157–161.)* Müllerian agenesis (or Mayer-Rokitansky-Kuster-Hauser syndrome) presents as amenorrhea with absence of a vagina. The incidence is approximately 1 in 10,000 female births. The karyotype is 46,XX. There is normal development of breasts, sexual hair, ovaries, tubes, and external genitalia. There are associated skeletal (12 percent) and urinary tract (33 percent) anomalies. Treatment generally consists of progressive vaginal dilatation or creation of an artificial vagina with split thickness skin grafts (McIndoe procedure). Testicular feminization or congenital androgen insensitivity syndrome is an X-linked recessive disorder with a karyotype of 46,XY. This accounts for 10 percent of all cases of primary amenorrhea. The patient presents with an absent uterus and blind vaginal canal. The amount of sexual hair is decreased. Although, there is a 25-percent incidence of malignant tumors in these patients, gonadectomy should be deferred until after full development is obtained. In other patients with a Y chromosome, gonadectomy should be performed as early as possible to prevent masculinization. Patients with gonadal dysgenesis would present with lack of secondary sexual characteristics. Patients with Klinefelter syndrome typically have a karyotype of 47,XXY and have a male phenotype. Genetic causes of primary amenorrhea in descending order of frequency are gonadal dysgenesis, müllerian agenesis, and testicular feminization.

365. The answer is A (1, 2, 3). *(Kase, pp 315–320.)* Anorexia nervosa is characterized by self-induced starvation and emaciation in the absence of organic disease. It is seen most commonly in adolescent girls and rarely occurs in boys. Most affected individuals have an obsessive-compulsive personality. It has been shown that the mean 24-hour cortisol concentration is twice normal because of increased circulation half-life and a decreased metabolic clearance rate. The daily cortisol production remains unchanged. These patients also have a low triiodothyronine (T_3) syndrome; both T_3 and thyroxine (T_4) are below normal values, with T_3 at a much lower level probably because of disturbance in the peripheral conversion of T_4 to T_3.

366. The answer is B (1, 3). *(Speroff, ed 3. pp 145–149.)* In the workup of primary amenorrhea, prolactin, TSH, and a progestational challenge test are the initial studies ordered. If patients are hyperprolactinemic or hypothyroid, appropriate therapy can then be initiated. FSH-LH and karyotype are occasionally necessary later in the evaluation of these patients. In all patients presenting with amenorrhea, pregnancy must be ruled out.

367. The answer is B (1, 3). *(Speroff, ed 3. p 156.)* Asherman syndrome is intrauterine synechia that usually follows a too-vigorous postpartum curettage. Affected women continue to ovulate, although they do not have menstrual bleeding; their basic body temperatures, therefore, are biphasic and normal. The diagnosis of Asherman syndrome is made by hysteroscopy or by hysterosalpingography. The etiology is not related to insertion of an intrauterine device (IUD), but IUDs have been utilized in treatment, because they separate the walls of the uterus after the adhesions are broken. However, a pediatric Foley catheter appears to be a better method of effecting the separation. After placement of the catheter, affected women should begin taking high doses of estrogen for 3 weeks a month, allowing the endometrium to regenerate.

368. The answer is E (all). *(Wilson, ed 7. pp 188–189.)* Postpartum panhypopituitarism is caused by hemorrhage in and subsequent necrosis of the pituitary gland, which is enlarged during pregnancy. Temporal arteritis and sickle cell anemia lead to panhypopituitarism by causing chronic vascular insufficiency of the pituitary gland. Hand-Schüller-Christian disease causes panhypopituitarism as a result of the infiltration of the gland by cholesterol-laden histiocytes. In the empty-sella syndrome, the pituitary gland becomes compressed within the sella. The pressure eventually leads to necrosis of the tissue, and the gland becomes nonfunctional.

369. The answer is B (1, 3). *(Wilson, ed 7. pp 1097–1101.)* Patients who have anorexia nervosa, a loss of appetite due to emotional reasons, show a striking loss of body mass on physical examination; patients who have panhypopituitarism, however, show marked wasting only infrequently. Axillary and pubic hair are not lost in patients affected by anorexia nervosa, because circulating steroid levels are maintained. Steroid levels in panhypopituitarism, on the other hand, are low, causing loss of axillary and pubic hair. In panhypopituitarism, the human growth hormone level is extremely low and thyroid activity is decreased significantly; these values are either normal or elevated in anorectic individuals.

370. The answer is A (1, 2, 3). *(Speroff, ed 3. p 225.)* Estrogen withdrawal bleeding, estrogen breakthrough bleeding, and progesterone breakthrough bleeding are mechanisms of dysfunctional uterine bleeding, which is defined as bleeding that does not occur according to a normal cycle. Progesterone withdrawal bleeding is the mechanism by which normal menstrual flow commences. A woman normally ovulates on day 14, and the corpus luteum begins producing progesterone. When progesterone production ceases about 14 days later, menstruation ensues.

371. The answer is C (2, 4). *(Speroff, ed 3. pp 207, 216–220.)* Treatment of hirsutism in many patients involves suppression of LH. This can be accomplished with progestational agents or birth-control pills. Patients should be informed that treatment is a slow process, taking from 6 months to 1 year before any change is noticed. In patients with predominantly adrenal androgen excess, treatment with dexamethasone can be tried. Progestational treatment will supress DHAS in most patients. Administration of spironolactone is a new approach in the treatment of hirsutism. It inhibits the ovarian biosynthesis of androgens and competes for the androgen receptor at the level of the hair follicle. Cimetidine and cyproterone acetate have also been used extensively in the treatment of hirsutism. Phenytoin, danazol, methyltestosterone, and anabolic agents can produce hirsutism.

372. The answer is E (all). *(Speroff, ed 3. pp 112–113.)* Premenstrual syndrome is a constellation of symptoms that occurs in a cyclic pattern, always in the same phase of the menstrual cycle. These symptoms usually occur 7 to 10 days before the onset of menses. Examples of symptoms reported include edema, mood swings, depression, irritability, breast tenderness, increased appetite, and cravings for sweets. The etiology is unclear, although endometriosis has been implicated. Besides the treatments listed in the question, therapy includes oral contraceptives, danazol, bromocriptine, evening primrose oil, and outdoor exercise. Controlled studies have been performed with most of the different treatment regimens with variable results. This is probably due to the difficulty in objective diagnosis.

373. The answer is A (1, 2, 3). *(Novak, ed 8. pp 817–829.)* Conservative measures for treating dysmenorrhea include heating pads, mild analgesics, sedatives or anti-spasmatic drugs, and outdoor exercise. In patients with dysmenorrhea there is a significantly higher-than-normal concentration of prostaglandins in the endometrium and menstrual fluid. Prostaglandin synthase inhibitors include indomethacin, naproxen, ibuprofen, and mefenamic acid. For patients with dysmenorrhea who are sexually active, oral contraceptives will provide needed protection from unwanted pregnancy and generally eleviate the dysmenorrhea.

374. The answer is E (all). *(Speroff, ed 3. pp 376–381.)* Delayed puberty is a rare condition, usually differentiated into hypergonadotropic hypogonadism or hypogonadotropic hypogonadism. The most common cause of hypergonadotropic hypogonadism is gonadal dysgenesis, i.e., the 45,X Turner syndrome. Hypogonadotropic hypogonadism can be seen in patients with hypothalamic pituitary or constitutional delays in development. Kallmann syndrome presents with amenorrhea, infantile sexual development, low gonadotropins, normal female karyotype, and the inability to perceive odors. In addition to those listed above, many other types of medical and nutritional problems can lead to this type of delayed development, e.g., malabsorption, diabetes, chronic illness, and regional ileitis.

375–379. The answers are: 375-D, 376-B, 377-A, 378-A, 379-C. *(Speroff, ed 3. pp 371–376.)* True sexual precocity in girls is characterized by elevated gonadotropin levels and a normal ovulatory pattern. It represents premature activation of a normally operating hypothalamus-pituitary relationship. Although it usually is idiopathic, true sexual precocity can arise from cerebral causes as well as from hypothyroidism, polyostotic fibrous dysplasia, neurofibromatosis, and other disorders.

In girls who have precocious pseudopuberty, the endocrine glands, usually under neoplastic influences, produce elevated amounts of estrogens (isosexual precocious pseudopuberty) or androgens (heterosexual precocious pseudopuberty.) Ovarian tumors appear to be the most common cause of isosexual precocious pseudopuberty; and some ovarian tumors, including dysgerminomas and choriocarcinomas, can produce so much gonadotropin that pregnancy tests are positive.

Incomplete sexual precocity, which usually is idiopathic, is characterized by only partial sexual maturity, such as premature thelarche, premature pubarche, or premature adrenarche. Incomplete sexual precocity can be accompanied by abnormal central-nervous-system function (e.g., mental deficiency).

In gonadotropin-producing tumors, high levels of gonadotropins, such as FSH, are produced with subsequent production of estrogen. Examples of these tumors are hepatoma, chorioepithelioma, and presacral tumors.

380–383. The answers are: 380-B, 381-D, 382-C, 383-A. *(Speroff, ed 3. pp 225–241, 478–481.)* Dysfunctional uterine bleeding is bleeding from the endometrium, independent of anatomic problems (e.g., pregnancy or fibroids, polyps, cancer, foreign bodies, or infection). In patients who are sexually active with anovulatory bleeding, optimal therapy would be oral contraceptive until the patient is ready to start a family. If the patient is not sexually active, cycling with a progestational agent 10 days out of each month would be appropriate. In an older patient with abnormal bleeding, endometrial sampling to rule out adenomatous hyperplasia or endometrial cancer is mandatory. Antiprostaglandins have been used, not only in young patients but in older patients, to decrease the amount of menstrual flow along with alleviating dysmenorrhea. An inadequate luteal phase is generally a result of decreased progesterone production by the corpus luteum. Treatment consists of either clomiphene or progesterone.

Pelvic Relaxation, Infections, Endometriosis, and Infertility

DIRECTIONS: Each question below contains five suggested responses. Select the **one best** response to each question.

384. Common problems occurring after a vaginal hysterectomy and anteroposterior repair for uterine prolapse include all the following EXCEPT

(A) stress urinary incontinence
(B) dyspareunia
(C) nonfistulous fecal incontinence
(D) enterocele
(E) vaginal vault prolapse

385. There are many different causes of urinary incontinence in the female. After stress incontinence, the most common cause of urinary leakage is

(A) detrusor dyssynergia
(B) unstable bladder
(C) unstable urethra
(D) urethral diverticulum
(E) overflow incontinence

386. Which is the most common sign of impending evisceration from a wound incision?

(A) Serous drainage
(B) Sanguineous drainage
(C) Serosanguineous drainage
(D) Abdominal pain with no drainage
(E) Abdominal contents in the wound

387. All the following statements regarding gonorrhea are true EXCEPT that

(A) most women infected with *Neisseria gonorrhoeae* are asymptomatic
(B) the definitive diagnosis for gonorrhea depends upon a positive culture
(C) at diagnosis a serologic test for syphilis should also be performed
(D) the usual reason for treatment failure is penicillin-resistant gonococci
(E) gonococcal infections resistant to both penicillin and spectinomycin should be treated with cefoxitin

388. The photomicrograph below shows a portion of uterine wall from a 43-year-old woman who has chronic pelvic pain and dysmenorrhea that is unresponsive to hormonal therapy. The most likely diagnosis is

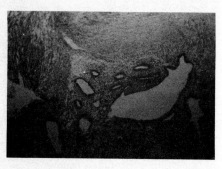

(A) endometriosis
(B) adenomyosis
(C) endometrial carcinoma
(D) ovarian carcinoma
(E) squamous cell carcinoma of the vulva

389. A woman has been anuric for the first 48 hours after undergoing abdominal hysterectomy. Bilateral ligation of the ureters is suspected. Which of the following therapeutic measures should first be ordered?

(A) Observation only
(B) Ureteral catheterization
(C) Rapid dialysis
(D) Transabdominal deligation
(E) Bilateral nephrostomy

390. All the following statements concerning endometriosis are true EXCEPT

(A) symptoms include pain, dysmenorrhea, and dyspareunia
(B) the most common site of implantation is the ovary
(C) there is a polygenic, multifactorial inheritance pattern
(D) there is an increased incidence of spontaneous abortions in patients with endometriosis
(E) endometriosis is a rare finding in black patients

391. Varicoceles are related to male infertility. All the following statements are true EXCEPT that

(A) varicoceles are found in approximately 15 percent of the general population
(B) the majority of varicoceles occur on the left side
(C) the size of the varix preoperatively correlates well with the prognosis of the success of surgery
(D) the most striking improvement with varicocele ligation is improvement in sperm motility
(E) the characteristic semen analysis associated with varicoceles shows the so-called stress pattern

392. An enterocele is best characterized by which of the following statements?

(A) It is not a true hernia
(B) It is a herniation of the bladder
floor into the vagina
(C) It is a prolapse of the uterus and
vaginal wall outside the body
(D) It is a protrusion of the pelvic peritoneal sac and vaginal wall into
the vagina
(E) It is a herniation of the rectal and
vaginal wall into the vagina

393. Asherman syndrome is associated
with infertility. All the following are
true EXCEPT that

(A) symptoms include amenorrhea or
hypomenorrhea
(B) patients are usually anovulatory
(C) diagnosis is made by hysterosalpingogram
(D) treatment consists of lysis of
adhesions
(E) prophylactic antibiotics are a wise
precaution for the surgical treatment of Asherman syndrome

394. All the following statements
about herpes genitalis are true EX-
CEPT that

(A) affected women may present with
urinary retention
(B) many affected women have accompanying trichomoniasis or
Haemophilus vaginalis vaginitis
(C) primary infections can be asymptomatic
(D) recurrent lesions tend to be disseminated and conspicuous
(E) use of tricyclic dyes can shorten
the clinical course

395. Risk factors in the development
of acute salpingitis include all the following EXCEPT

(A) an age of 15 to 24 years
(B) oral contraceptives
(C) presence of an intrauterine device
(D) multiple sex partners
(E) previous gonorrhea or salpingitis

396. All the following are effective
treatment regimens for acute salpingitis
EXCEPT

(A) cefoxitin plus doxycycline
(B) clindamycin plus gentamicin
(C) metronidazole plus doxycycline
(D) penicillin plus gentamicin
(E) ampicillin, gentamicin, and clinda-
mycin

397. Indications for hospitalization of
a patient with salpingitis include all the
following EXCEPT

(A) temperature greater than 38°C
(B) presence of an adnexal mass
(C) presence of intracellular diplococci
on Gram stain
(D) peritonitis
(E) coexisting pregnancy

398. All the following statements
about endometriosis are true EXCEPT
that

(A) malignant changes are rare
(B) a diagnosis is often established by
history and physical examination
(C) it is more common in women in
their reproductive years than in
postmenopausal women
(D) affected women may present with
infertility
(E) the most common site of involvement is the ovary

399. All the following statements about danazol are true EXCEPT that

(A) danazol is a progestational derivative of testosterone
(B) danazol will inhibit basal gonadotropin levels
(C) the endometrial response to danazol is atrophy
(D) prompt return of menses and ovulation is noted when danazol is discontinued
(E) one should delay pregnancy at least 3 months after danazol therapy

400. All the following are causes of vaginal discharge in young children EXCEPT

(A) mycoplasma
(B) *Enterobius vermicularis*
(C) foreign bodies
(D) *N. gonorrhoeae*
(E) mycotic infection

401. At the present time therapy for women who have mild to moderate endometriosis can consist of all the following EXCEPT

(A) progestins
(B) dexamethasone
(C) danazol
(D) gonadotropin releasing hormone
(E) conservative surgery

DIRECTIONS: Each question below contains four suggested responses of which **one or more** is correct. Select

A	if	**1, 2, and 3**	are correct
B	if	**1 and 3**	are correct
C	if	**2 and 4**	are correct
D	if	**4**	is correct
E	if	**1, 2, 3, and 4**	are correct

402. Possible sequelae of acute salpingitis include

(1) infertility
(2) ectopic pregnancies
(3) chronic pelvic pain
(4) adhesions

403. Etiological factors important in the development of genital prolapse include

(1) poor tissue strength
(2) chronic straining at bowel movements
(3) menopause
(4) childbirth trauma

404. Organisms commonly involved in the development of acute salpingitis include

(1) *N. gonorrhoeae*
(2) peptostreptococci and peptococci
(3) *B. fragilis*
(4) *Clostridium perfringens*

405. For couples in the United States between the ages of 18 and 28 years engaging in unprotected intercourse four times per week, which of the following conception rates should be anticipated?

(1) Fifty percent will be pregnant by 4 months
(2) Sixty percent will be pregnant in 6 months
(3) Eighty percent will conceive in 1 year
(4) During the first year, the chance of conception per monthly cycle is 15 percent

406. If ureteral injury is recognized at the time of surgery, which of the following procedures could be recommended?

(1) A longitudinal slit should be made in the ureter below the injury and a polyethylene tube threaded into the bladder
(2) If the ureter is not severed, the site of injury should be drained intraperitoneally
(3) If the ureter is severed, ureteroureteral anastomosis should be attempted, regardless of the location of the injury
(4) If possible, the severed ureter should be implanted into the bladder

SUMMARY OF DIRECTIONS

A	B	C	D	E
1,2,3 only	1,3 only	2,4 only	4 only	All are correct

407. Luteal-phase defect is associated with faulty ovulation. Which of the following studies performed in the second half of the menstrual cycle would be helpful in making a diagnosis?

(1) Serum progesterone levels
(2) Urine pregnanetriol levels
(3) Endometrial biopsy
(4) Serum luteinizing hormone levels

408. There are several serologic tests for syphilis. True statements about nontreponemal tests and specific antitreponemal antibody tests include which of the following?

(1) The nontreponemal test should become positive within 7 to 14 days after chancre formation
(2) When successful treatment is employed early enough, the nontreponemal test will usually return to negative
(3) FTA is the most commonly used specific antitreponemal antibody test
(4) FTA remains positive indefinitely after treatment

409. During gynecological surgery, operative injuries to the ureter occur

(1) more frequently in association with vaginal rather than abdominal hysterectomy
(2) only rarely if periureteral tissue is dissected carefully
(3) most commonly when the ureter lies between the anterior vaginal wall and the base of the bladder
(4) often as a result of hasty reclamping of vessel clamps or ligatures

410. Histological features that are diagnostic for endometriosis include

(1) endometrial glands
(2) evidence of hemorrhage
(3) endometrial stroma
(4) decidual reaction in the surrounding tissue

411. The x-ray shown below reveals which of the following?

(1) Cornual obstruction
(2) Distended tubes
(3) Bilateral spill
(4) Bilateral hydrosalpinx

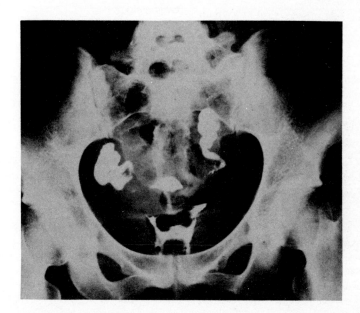

412. Retrograde menstruation is the most accepted explanation of the etiology of endometriosis. Which of the following statements may be cited as evidence for this theory?

(1) Inversion of the cervix of a monkey into the peritoneal cavity can cause endometriosis
(2) Endometrial tissue can be cultured successfully
(3) Menstrual blood can come from the ends of the fallopian tubes of some women
(4) Endometrial glands can arise from coelomic epithelium

SUMMARY OF DIRECTIONS

A	B	C	D	E
1,2,3 only	1,3 only	2,4 only	4 only	All are correct

413. Treatments commonly employed for women who have the vulvar lesions shown below include

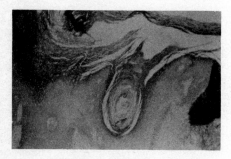

(1) podophyllum
(2) trichloroacidic acid
(3) laser therapy
(4) simple vulvectomy

414. Which of the following conditions can predispose to vaginal infection with *Candida albicans*?

(1) Pregnancy
(2) Antibiotic therapy
(3) Adrenocorticosteroid therapy
(4) Presence of an intrauterine device

415. In the treatment of stress urinary incontinence, the disadvantages of the Marshall-Marchetti-Krantz procedure compared with other surgical alternatives include

(1) urinary retention
(2) increased incidence of urinary tract infections
(3) high failure rate
(4) osteitis pubis

416. For the objective diagnosis of stress urinary incontinence, which of the following tests may be performed?

(1) Urine culture
(2) Urethrocystoscopy
(3) Cystometrography
(4) Physical examination including neurologic evaluation, Q-tip test, and stress test

417. True statements concerning fecal
incontinence include that

(1) in the presence of traumatic injury
to the rectal sphincter, the patient
will have a high degree of continence provided the puborectalis
muscle is intact
(2) diabetic patients are unlikely to experience fecal incontinence
(3) obstetrical trauma is one of the
most common causes of fecal incontinence
(4) therapy with bulk-forming agents
and antispasmodics (e.g., Lomotil
and Metamucil) will aggravate the
fecal incontinence problem

DIRECTIONS: Each group of questions below consists of lettered headings followed by a set of numbered items. For each numbered item select the **one** lettered heading with which it is **most** closely associated. Each lettered heading may be used **once, more than once, or not at all.**

Questions 418–421

Match each infertility test with the appropriate time for it to be done in a 28-day cycle.

(A) Day 2
(B) Day 8
(C) Day 14
(D) Day 24
(E) Day 28

418. Hysterosalpingography

419. Postcoital testing

420. Endometrial biopsy

421. Serum progesterone

Questions 422–425

For each patient below, select the appropriate antibiotic.

(A) Tetracycline
(B) Procaine penicillin
(C) Metronidazole
(D) Benzathine penicillin
(E) Spectinomycin

422. A 35-year-old woman has recently been diagnosed as having primary syphilis

423. A 23-year-old woman with acute salpingitis being treated with gentamicin and clindamycin is not responding. Culture of the cervix was positive for chlamydia

424. A 34-year-old patient with a tubo-ovarian abscess was started on penicillin and gentamicin. Purulent material aspirated from the cul-de-sac has revealed *B. fragilis*. The patient has failed to respond

425. A 28-year-old woman has a penicillinase-producing *N. gonorrhoeae*

Questions 426–429

For each description that follows, select the operative procedure with which it is most likely to be associated.

(A) Salpingoplasty
(B) Salpingostomy
(C) Salpingolysis
(D) Fimbriolysis
(E) Uterotubal implantation

426. Forming a patent entry site in the fundal portion of the uterus and attaching the oviduct

427. Cutting adhesions causing conglutination of the distal end of the oviduct

428. Cutting adhesions around the uterine tube

429. Opening up a previously formed hydrosalpinx

Questions 430–434

Match the descriptions below with the appropriate infectious agent or condition.

(A) *Candida albicans*
(B) *Trichomonas vaginalis*
(C) *Neisseria gonorrhoeae*
(D) *Corynebacterium vaginale (Haemophilus vaginalis)*
(E) Atrophic (senile) vaginitis

430. A frequent cause of nonspecific vaginitis

431. Diabetes mellitus may be a predisposing factor

432. Typically produces a frothy discharge

433. Typically produces a grossly recognizable, punctate hemorrhagic vaginal mucosa ("strawberry spots")

434. Treatment with an estrogen cream may be effective

Pelvic Relaxation, Infections, Endometriosis, and Infertility

Answers

384. The answer is C. *(Mattingly, ed 6. pp 547–561, 569–593.)* Many patients who have uterine prolapse or a large protuberant cystocele will be continent because of urethral obstruction. At times, patients need to reduce the prolapse in order to void. During surgical repair, if the urethral vesical junction is not properly elevated, urinary incontinence may result. Dyspareunia can be caused by shortening of the vagina, or constriction at the introitus. If the vaginal vault is not properly suspended and the uterosacral ligaments plicated, vaginal vault prolapse or enterocele may occur at a later date. Fecal incontinence is not a complication of vaginal hysterectomy with repair. It may occur, however, if a fistula is formed through unrecognized damage to the rectal mucosa.

385. The answer is B. *(Ostergard, ed 2. pp 69–78, 363–369.)* The most common cause of urinary incontinence is incompetence of the urethral sphincter or genuine stress incontinence. Stress incontinence is the involuntary loss of urine when intravesical pressure exceeds the maximum urethral pressure, in the absence of detrusor activity. The other major cause of incontinence is the unstable bladder. An unstable bladder is the occurrence of involuntary, uninhibited detrusor contractions of greater than 15 cm of water pressure, with simultaneous urethral relaxation. The incidence of patients with incontinence due to an unstable bladder can vary from 8.7 to 63 percent of patients presenting with incontinence. Other causes of urinary incontinence include overflow secondary to urinary retention, congenital abnormalities, infections, and fistulas. Detrusor dyssynergia implies that when the patient has an uninhibited detrusor contraction, there is simultaneous contraction of the urethral or periurethral striated muscle (normally there is urethral relaxation with a detrusor contraction). This is generally seen in patients with neurologic lesions. Urethral diverticula classically present with dribbling incontinence after voiding.

386. The answer is C. *(Mattingly, ed 6. pp 171–174.)* Serosanguineous drainage occurs very frequently before evisceration from the incision. Drainage can be accompanied by pain or by the feeling that something is "giving way." Serous or sanguineous drainage often is noted postoperatively and usually suggests involvement of the superficial wound.

387. The answer is D. *(Kase, p 604.)* Gonococcus can persist asymptomatically in women for weeks to months. Although gonorrhea may be suspected clinically, a positive culture should be obtained before informing the patient that she is infected. There is an increased incidence of syphilis in women with gonorrhea, and this should be evaluated. The usual reason for treatment failure is reinfection; therefore, it should be stressed that both partners should be treated. Cefoxitin is the treatment of choice for gonorrhea resistant to penicillin and spectinomycin.

388. The answer is B. *(Blaustein, ed 2. pp 297–299.)* The histological and historical evidence presented in the question suggests adenomyosis. Adenomyosis is defined as endometrial tissue outside of the endometrial cavity and confined to the uterine wall. Tufts of endometrial tissue can be surrounded by areas of smooth muscle (myometrium), as in the accompanying photomicrograph. Endometriosis is defined as endometrial tissue outside of the uterus. Because the lesion shown is certainly benign, ovarian carcinoma and carcinoma of the vulva are ruled out. Women who have adenomyosis suffer from chronic pelvic pain and dysmenorrhea, usually associated with an enlarged uterus. A diagnosis is rarely made clinically and usually depends on pathological examination.

389. The answer is B. *(Mattingly, ed 6. pp 331–337.)* Bilateral ureteral obstruction, if unrecognized or unrelieved, can cause death in 7 to 10 days. Once the presence of bilateral ureteral obstruction is suspected, bilateral ureteral catheters should be passed in order to demonstrate and, if possible, overcome the obstructions. If obstruction persists, bilateral nephrostomy should be performed; if, 6 to 8 weeks later, the obstructions still cannot be overcome, ureteral surgery should be undertaken.

390. The answer is E. *(Mattingly, ed 6. pp 260–284.)* Symptoms seen in patients presenting with endometriosis include lower abdominal pain, usually aggravated premenstrually or menstrually, dysmenorrhea in up to 50 percent of patients, dyspareunia especially if there is involvement of the uterosacral ligaments, and dysfunctional uterine bleeding. Investigators find that approximately 30 percent of patients presenting with infertility have endometriosis as the predominant cause. The most common site of implantation is the ovary; however, implants can be found essentially in any location in the lower pelvis. There appears to be an increased incidence of endometriosis in first-degree relatives. Patients with endometriosis have been reported to have an increased incidence of spontaneous abortions. Although, at one time it was believed that endometriosis was rare in black patients, recent data suggest that this is not the case.

391. The answer is C. *(Kase, pp 438–439.)* The incidence of varicoceles in the general population is about 15 percent, but 40 percent of males with infertility are found to have varicoceles. Because of the anatomy and physiology, varicoceles are more likely to occur on the left side. There is no correlation between the size of the varix and fertility prognosis. The characteristic "stress pattern" seen with varicoceles is decreased number of sperm, decreased motility, and increased abnormal forms.

392. The answer is D. *(Mattingly, ed 6. pp 575–589.)* An enterocele is the protrusion of the pelvic peritoneal sac and the vaginal wall into the vagina. It is a true hernia, and it may be either congenital or associated with a uterine prolapse. Enteroceles can also occur following vaginal hysterectomy if the cul-de-sac is not adequately obliterated. Most commonly, patients with enteroceles complain of a mass protruding from the vagina when they strain, cough, sneeze, or perform other activities associated with the Valsalva maneuver—that is, activities causing pressure (by exhalation) against a closed glottis. Also, if intestines are present in the herniated sac, local discomfort will probably result.

393. The answer is B. *(Kase, p 457.)* Ovulation is not affected in Asherman syndrome. Because of the decreased amount of functional endometrium, hypomenorrhea or amenorrhea is common. The best diagnostic study is the hysterosalpingogram under fluoroscopy. Hysteroscopy with lysis of adhesions is the treatment of choice. Prophylactic antibiotics may improve success rates.

394. The answer is D. *(Romney, ed 2. pp 924–925.)* The symptoms of primary herpes genitalis, which include blisters, ulcers, pain, and urinary retention, are often severe and may persist for several weeks. Several studies have shown that a number of women who show no signs of herpes genitalis have antibodies to herpes simplex virus type 2, the causative agent of the disease; this finding indicates that these women have had previous, asymptomatic infections. Recurrent infections, which occur commonly, are localized and often hard to identify. Treatment of herpetic lesions is being attempted with many agents. The most promising of those already approved by the FDA is acyclovir. Many newer agents are still under investigation.

395. The answer is B. *(Mattingly, ed 6. pp 287–298.)* Acute salpingitis or pelvic inflammatory disease (PID) is a disease predominantly of nulliparous, young women. The IUD increases the risk of developing salpingitis three- to fivefold. The number of sexual partners and the incidence of sexually transmitted disease in a population also influence the development of PID. Oral contraceptives are felt to have a protective effect on developing infections; the risk is 30 to 90 percent that of nonusers. Condoms, diaphragms, and chemical barriers also provide protection from disease.

396. The answer is D. *(Monif, ed 2. pp 553–558.)* Treatment regimens for acute salpingitis should include agents active against gonorrhea and anaerobic organisms (e.g., *Bacteroides fragilis*). Doxycycline has been added to many regimens to cover chlamydial infection. There is no single-agent therapy active against the entire spectrum of pathogens. The combination of penicillin and gentamicin is inadequate because it fails to cover adequately anaerobic organisms and chlamydia.

397. The answer is C. *(Mattingly, ed 6. p 293.)* Patients should be hospitalized if they have a temperature, peritonitis, inability to tolerate oral medication, pregnancy, presence of a pelvic mass, an IUD, or failure to respond to out-patient therapy. The presence of intracellular diplococci or even proven culture of *N. gonorrhoeae* should not influence therapeutic management. The presence of gonorrhea in the cervix or vagina does not necessarily imply that pelvic inflammatory disease exists. Many patients present with asymptomatic gonorrhea.

398. The answer is B. *(Romney, ed 2. pp 932–933, 938–940.)* Endometriosis, which most commonly involves the ovaries, is a disease of women in their reproductive years, especially between the ages of 30 and 40 years. The disease is usually benign. The definitive diagnosis of endometriosis rarely can be established short of surgery or diagnostic laparoscopy. Diagnosis is aided by the presence of vulvar, vaginal, or cervical lesions, which can be biopsied; palpable cul-de-sac nodules; and a history of dysmenorrhea and infertility.

399. The answer is B. *(Kase, p 480.)* Danazol is a progestational compound derived from testosterone. It induces a pseudomenopause but does not alter basal gonadotropin levels. It appears to act as an antiestrogen and will cause endometrial atrophy. Cyclic menses return almost immediately upon danazol withdrawal. It is felt that the endometrium is poorly developed with danazol use and that three menstrual cycles should be allowed to go by before conceiving so as to avoid a higher risk of spontaneous abortion and other problems of poor implantation.

400. The answer is A. *(Huffman, ed 2. pp 121–140.)* Infections and inflammation of the vulva account for 85 to 90 percent of all genital problems in premenarcheal girls. Although perhaps the largest numbers seen are of nonspecific vulvovaginitis, in 5 percent of patients foreign bodies of all types are found. *Enterobius vermicularis* or pinworms are responsible for many intractable vulvovaginal infections and a Scotch tape test should be one of the first diagnostic studies performed on these children. Mycotic infections with *Candida* are seen in women of all ages. *N. gonorrhoeae* can cause severe inflammation and discharge in young children. At this time, there is no evidence that mycoplasmas cause premenarcheal vaginitis.

401.   The answer is B. *(Kase, pp 479–481, 515–518.)* One of the first medical treatments for endometriosis was the uninterrupted administration of high-dose birth-control pills for prolonged periods of time. Today this regimen is seldom given. Progestin therapy can lead to subjective and objective improvement in patients with endometriosis. Problems include break-through bleeding and depression. Overall, however, the side effects of progestin therapy are less than those with other treatments. Progestin therapy is generally reserved for patients who do not desire fertility. Danazol is an isoxazol derivative of 17-alpha-ethinyl testosterone and has been characterized as a pseudomenopausal treatment for endometriosis. Side effects include weight gain, edema, decreased breast size, acne, and other menopausal symptoms. GNRH agonist is the most recent addition to our armamentarium of drugs active against endometriosis. It indeed produces a medical oophorectomy. Collaborative studies are now being performed to see if fertility rates and cures for endometriosis are similar to those of other medications. At the present time, conservative surgery compares favorably with danazol administration in the management of mild to moderate endometriosis. Surgery is definitely indicated in patients with severe disease, those who fail hormonal therapy, or in the older infertile patient. Dexamethasone is not a treatment for endometriosis.

402.   The answer is E (all). *(Blaustein, ed 2. pp 397–398.)* Common sequelae of pelvic inflammatory disease are chronic pain, dyspareunia, adhesions, pyosalpinges, tuboovarian abscess, ectopic pregnancies, and infertility. After one episode of pelvic inflammatory disease the percentage of patients who become infertile is estimated at approximately 11 percent. With three or more episodes, the percentage of infertile patients increases to 54 percent. There is a six- to tenfold increase in ectopic pregnancies after salpingitis.

403.   The answer is E (all). *(Novak, ed 8. pp 351–376.)* All the factors mentioned in the question are commonly seen in patients with genital problems. Undoubtedly, the most important factor is the actual quality of the tissue itself. In black patients and in Chinese there is a much lower incidence of uterine prolapse and enterocele formation in comparison with whites. Any factors that increase abdominal pressure can aggravate or further deteriorate the prolapse. Although the actual number of deliveries is probably not important, traumatic deliveries, especially those in which the rectal sphincter is lacerated or improperly repaired, have been associated with pelvic relaxation.

404. The answer is A (1, 2, 3). *(Blaustein, ed 2. pp 397–398.)* Gonococcal infection in patients with salpingitis has been reported in 33 to 81 percent of patients. Gonorrhea has been cultured from the peritoneal cavity in 6 to 70 percent of these patients. Anaerobic bacteria such as peptostreptococci, peptococci, and bacteroides have demonstrated that salpingitis is a polymicrobial disease. Scandanavian studies report a high incidence of chlamydial infection. *Clostridium perfringens*, at one time, was a cause of septic shock in patients following illegal abortions. It is rarely seen today.

405. The answer is E (all). *(Kase, p 426.)* These figures are used when investigating a couple for potential fertility. Approximately 20 percent of couples attempting pregnancy for 1 year will be unsuccessful. Half of those will spontaneously conceive during the second year. Half of those remaining, or approximately 5 percent, will benefit from specific therapy.

406. The answer is D (4). *(Mattingly, ed 6. pp 325–344.)* Following an injury to the ureter during surgery, a drain should be placed extraperitoneally. If a polyethylene catheter is inserted, it should be placed above the site of injury so that urine is drained before arrival at the site of injury. Ureteroureteral anastomosis should be done only if reimplantation into the bladder is not feasible. Implanting a severed ureter into the bladder is the procedure of choice.

407. The answer is B (1, 3). *(Speroff, ed 3. pp 478–482.)* A short luteal phase is defined as ovulation with poor production of progesterone in the second half of the cycle. Progesterone levels at that time of less than 7 ng/ml are diagnostic. Endometrial biopsy also is crucial to the diagnosis of this defect, because the endometrium will be out of phase with the time of cycle. For example, a biopsy taken on day 26 of the cycle will resemble endometrium of day 24 because of decreased progesterone stimulation. Pregnanetriol is a breakdown product of 17-hydroxyprogesterone, and levels are not helpful in diagnosing this condition. Determination of the level of pregnanediol, which is a metabolic product of progesterone excreted in the urine, is a helpful test. Serum luteinizing hormone levels have no correlation with the presence of a luteal-phase defect.

408. The answer is E (all). *(Kase, p 605.)* Current nontreponemal tests include RPR and VDRL. These tests are useful for screening. They become positive 1 to 2 weeks after chancre formation and remain positive indefinitely if untreated. The fluorescent treponemal antibody absorbtion test (FTA-ABS) is the most commonly used antitreponemal test. FTA does become positive earlier than RPR and will remain positive indefinitely even after treatment. One cannot follow FTA titers as a measure of cure or reinfection.

409. The answer is D (4). *(Mattingly, ed 6. pp 325–344.)* Operative injuries to the ureter are associated more commonly with abdominal hysterectomy than vaginal hysterectomy. The most common site of injury occurs near the region of the uterine vessels. Because the blood supply to the ureter arises from the periureteral tissue, dissection should be avoided; even careful dissection results in a significant percentage of ureteral injuries, and the incidence of fistula formation is increased if the blood supply is compromised. Slippage of vessels from clamps or ligatures can lead to ureteral injury if the vessels are reclamped hastily in an effort to stop the resultant bleeding.

410. The answer is A (1, 2, 3). *(Blaustein, ed 2. p 468.)* In view of the importance of accuracy in diagnosing endometriosis, strict, definitive criteria must be used. The triad of histological findings that is diagnostic for endometriosis consists of the presence of endometrial glands and endometrial stroma and evidence of recent or old hemorrhage. In women who are pregnant or who are receiving certain forms of hormonal therapy, a significant decidual reaction may be seen; this feature, however, is by no means diagnostic for endometriosis.

411. The answer is C (2, 4). *(Kistner, ed 4. pp 425–427.)* The x-ray presented reveals bilateral hydrosalpinx and distended tubes; no spill is noted at the fimbriated extremity. These findings are suggestive of chronic pelvic inflammatory disease. Both cornual areas appear normal, and there is no spill into the peritoneal cavity.

412. The answer is A (1, 2, 3). *(Speroff, ed 3. p 494.)* Retrograde menstruation is currently believed to be a major cause of endometriosis. Supporting this belief are the following findings: inversion of the uterine cervix into the peritoneal cavity can cause the monkey to develop endometriosis; endometrial tissue is viable outside the uterus; and blood can issue from the ends of the fallopian tubes of some women during menstruation. The fact that endometrial implants can occur in the lung implies that lymphatic or vascular routes of spread of the disease also are possible. Another theory of the etiology of endometriosis entails the conversion of coelomic epithelium into glands resembling those of the endometrium.

413. The answer is A (1, 2, 3). *(Kase, pp 614–615.)* The lesions shown in the figure accompanying the question are condyloma acuminatum, also known as the venereal wart. This is a squamous lesion caused by the papilloma virus. The lesion reveals a tree-like growth microscopically with a mantle that shows marked acanthosis and parakeratosis. The treatment is local excision, cryosurgery, or podophyllum, trichloroacidic acid, or laser therapy. For intractable condyloma of the vagina, 5-fluorouracil can be employed. Vulvectomy is rarely indicated. A strong relationship between condyloma and cervical interepithelial neoplasia / cervical carcinoma has recently been demonstrated.

414. The answer is A (1, 2, 3). *(Kase, pp 595–597.)* Pregnancy is associated with an increase in the incidence of monilial infections, probably because of an increase in glycogen content in the vaginal mucosa. Antibiotic therapy clearly increases the likelihood of candidiasis (moniliasis), perhaps because it eliminates susceptible bacteria that compete with *Candida* for available nutrients. Steroid therapy may involve inhibition of catabolic-enzyme release. No association exists between the use of intrauterine devices and a predisposition toward monilial infections.

415. The answer is D (4). *(Ostergard, ed 2. pp 479–493.)* There are many procedures that will provide successful correction of stress urinary incontinence. One of the abdominal procedures that successfully cures stress incontinence is the Marshall-Marchetti-Krantz (MMK) procedure. This involves the attachment of the periurethral tissue to the symphysis pubis. In approximately 3 percent of those patients undergoing the procedure, the debilitating condition of osteitis pubis will develop. An alternative—the Burch procedure—was, therefore, introduced; this involves the attachment of the periurethral tissue to Cooper's ligament. The incidences of urinary retention, recurrent urinary tract infections, and failure are essentially the same in the MMK and Burch procedures. Other procedures commonly employed in the treatment of stress incontinence are the anterior repair and needle urethropexy (Stamey-Pererya procedure). The traditional anterior repair, or Kelly plication, has a 5-year failure rate of approximately 50 percent. The initial cure rate (90 percent) of the Stamey-Pererya procedure appears to equal that of the Burch procedure.

416. The answer is E (all). *(Ostergard, ed 2. pp 45–58.)* One of the initial steps in the evaluation of patients with urinary incontinence is a urine culture. In many cases, symptoms and abnormal urodynamics will disappear after appropriate therapy. Urethrocystoscopy allows the physician to evaluate for the presence of urethral diverticula, urethritis, fistulas, and descent of the urethral vesicle junction. Since history alone is inadequate in diagnosing patients with an unstable bladder, a cystometrogram is mandatory in all patients considered as candidates for surgical correction of stress incontinence. The Q-tip test allows the physician to evaluate whether an anatomic defect is present (all surgical procedures designed to correct stress incontinence work by decreasing urethral mobility). The stress test provides the physician with objective evidence that, indeed, the patient does have urinary leakage.

417. The answer is B (1, 3). *(Mattingly, ed 6. pp 669–687.)* The most common cause of fecal incontinence is obstetrical trauma and inadequate repair. The rectal sphincter can be completely lacerated, but as long as the patients retain a functional puborectalis sling, a high degree of continence will be maintained. Generally, the patients are continent of form stool and not of flatus. Other causes include senility, CNS disease, rectal prolapse, diarrhea, and inflammation. Approximately 20 percent of all diabetics will complain of fecal incontinence. Therapy for fecal incontinence includes bulk and antispasmodic agents, especially in those patients presenting with diarrhea. All caffeinated beverages should be stopped. Biofeedback and electrical stimulation of the rectal sphincter are other possible conservative treatment modalities.

418–421. The answers are: 418-B, 419-C, 420-D, 421-D. *(Kase, pp 429–430.)* Hysterosalpingography should be performed sufficiently after menses to avoid retrograde movement of menstrual fluid through the tubes and sufficiently before ovulation so as not to interfere with possible conception or implantation. Postcoital testing is best done around ovulation to take advantage of optimal cervical mucus. Endometrial biopsy and serum progesterone are used to document ovulation and are best done between days 24 and 26 of the cycle.

422–425. The answers are: 422-D, 423-A, 424-C, 425-E. *(Monif, ed 2. pp 553–558.)* The treatment for primary syphilis is benzathine penicillin, 2.4 million units, IM. For those patients who are allergic to penicillin, tetracycline may be given. In a patient with acute salpingitis with culture-proven chlamydia who does not respond to conventional therapy, tetracycline should be added. Drugs active against *B. fragilis* include cefoxitin, clindamycin, metronidazole, and chloramphenicol. Many feel that patients presenting with pelvic inflammatory disease should be given a drug that has anaerobic coverage and that the regimen of pencillin and gentamicin is not adequate. Uncomplicated gonorrheal infections are generally treated with oral tetracycline, amoxicillin/ampicillin, or aqueous procaine penicillin. In patients with penicillinase-producing *N. gonorrhoeae*, spectinomycin 2 g IM is given in a single injection. An alternative medication is cefoxitin. Spectinomycin and cefoxitin are ineffective in pharyngeal infections.

426–429. The answers are: 426-E, 427-D, 428-C, 429-B. *(Sciarra, ed 51, vol 1, chap 74, pp 1–18.)* Salpingolysis, salpingoplasty, and uterotubal implantation are the major surgical techniques used by tubal surgeons. A salpingolysis is merely the cutting of adhesions surrounding the fallopian tube. Salpingoplasty, which is performed on the fimbriated end of the tube, is divided into two parts: fimbriolysis, which is a simple cutting of adhesions causing the fimbria to conglutinate in the midline, and salpingostomy, which is creation of an opening in tubes that were completely closed with hydrosalpinx, usually secondary to infection. On occasion, the tube is occluded at the cornual area, which must be excised, and a new opening into the uterus must be created; this procedure is uterotubal implantation. These procedures are commonly used to correct infertility problems related to lack of tubal patency or mobility interfering with ovum pickup/transport. Predisposing factors include endometriosis, pelvic inflammatory disease, appendicitis, and prior tubal ligation.

430–434. The answers are: 430-D, 431-A, 432-B, 433-B, 434-E. *(Sciarra, ed 51, vol 1, chap 24, pp 8–9; chap 26, pp 1–6.)* Many cases of nonspecific vaginitis are caused by *Corynebacterium vaginale*. These women usually complain of a characteristic malodorous, grayish vaginal discharge. On wet mounts, the diagnosis is made by visualizing the "clue cells," which are epithelial cells with large numbers of adherent coccobacilli. The recommended treatment is ampicillin, although vaginal sulfa creams are also effective.

Besides diabetes mellitus, other predisposing factors of candidiasis include pregnancy, the use of antibiotics, immunosuppressive medications, and possibly oral contraceptives. Affected individuals usually complain of severe pruritus and thick, cheese-like vaginal discharge. Wet mounts show characteristic yeast cells and hyphae. The primary mode of treatment is the vaginal application of an antifungal agent, such as nystatin.

Trichomonas vaginalis classically gives rise to a yellowish, frothy discharge, which is foul smelling and causes pruritus. The pathognomonic "strawberry spots," which consist of punctate hemorrhagic spots on the vaginal mucosa, can sometimes be seen. The diagnosis is made by observing the characteristic motile protozoan on wet mounts. The mainstay of treatment is oral metronidazole, either in a single dose of 2 g or 250 mg three times a day for 7 to 10 days. Metronidazole has a disulfiram-like effect, and women taking it should refrain from consumption of alcohol. Vaginal suppositories of clotrimazole, 100 mg once a day for 7 days, are also effective and are preferred by some because of carcinogenicity associated with rodents treated with metronidazole.

Postmenopausal women who present with symptoms like itching, irritation secondary to dryness, and dyspareunia often have atrophic (senile) vaginitis. Owing to the lack of estrogen, the vaginal mucosa becomes very thin and easily irritable. This condition responds well to either oral intake of estrogen or local application of estrogen creams.

The Bartholin's glands, endocervical glands, and fallopian tubes can all be infected by *N. gonorrhoeae*, but an infection of the vaginal mucosa is uncommon.

Benign and Malignant Neoplasms

DIRECTIONS: Each question below contains five suggested responses. Select the **one best** response to each question.

435. Which of the following statements regarding endometrioid carcinoma of the ovary is true?

(A) It accounts for the majority of epithelial ovarian carcinomas
(B) Malignant transformation of ovarian endometriosis has been demonstrated
(C) Squamous differentiation is uncommon
(D) It is indistinguishable from adenocarcinoma of endometrial origin
(E) Approximately 80 percent of endometrioid ovarian carcinomas are accompanied by ovarian endometriosis

436. In stage II carcinoma of the endometrium

(A) the length of the uterine cavity is less than 8 cm
(B) the corpus and the cervix are involved
(C) there is extension to the parametrium
(D) there is extension to the ovaries
(E) there is metastasis to the bladder

437. The primary mode of treatment for endometrial carcinoma confined to the uterine corpus is

(A) external beam radiation
(B) intracavitary radium
(C) hysterectomy
(D) chemotherapy
(E) progestin therapy

438. Fractional dilatation and curettage reveals endometrial carcinoma involving the cervix. This finding is

(A) of no prognostic significance
(B) of some prognostic significance but does not require change in management
(C) significant only if the cervical tumor is clinically obvious
(D) significant even if the disease is present only microscopically
(E) a contraindication for hysterectomy

439. The most common sarcoma of the uterus is

(A) endometrial stromal sarcoma
(B) carcinosarcoma
(C) leiomyosarcoma
(D) mixed mesodermal sarcoma
(E) rhabdomyosarcoma

440. Mixed mesodermal tumors of the uterus can be described by which of the following statements?

(A) They are more common than previously assumed and constitute about 17 to 18 percent of uterine malignancies
(B) Microscopic examination may reveal the presence of bone, cartilage, muscle, or other elements
(C) Their development has been associated with maternal intake of estrogen during pregnancy
(D) The 5-year survival rate is quite good (approximately 80 percent)
(E) They are not known to occur before the menopausal years

441. All the following statements are true of uterine leiomyoma EXCEPT

(A) it is three to nine times more common in white than black women
(B) it does not appear to occur before menarche
(C) on pathologic examination various forms of degeneration are seen
(D) common presenting complaints include abnormal bleeding and pressure symptoms
(E) surgery is generally indicated when the uterus is larger than 12 weeks size

442. All the following statements regarding ovarian cancer are true EXCEPT that

(A) it is the most common gynecological cancer
(B) it has the highest mortality among the common gynecological cancers
(C) it tends to be asymptomatic until it has reached an advanced stage
(D) its development may be influenced by environmental, cultural, or socioeconomic factors
(E) Papanicolaou (Pap) smears are ineffective for routine diagnostic screening

443. A 45-year-old woman has undergone a total abdominal hysterectomy and bilateral salpingo-oophorectomy for stage II serous carcinoma of the ovary. The most effective postoperative radiotherapeutic treatment of this woman would be

(A) pelvic irradiation
(B) vaginal radium insertion and pelvic irradiation
(C) whole-abdomen irradiation
(D) whole-abdomen and pelvic irradiation
(E) intraperitoneal radioisotope therapy

444. Which of the following statements best describes adenomyosis?

(A) It is a serious disease of the endometrium
(B) It is more common in nulliparas
(C) Patients frequently present with hypermenorrhea, acquired dysmenorrhea, and a slightly enlarged, tender uterus
(D) It most often occurs postmenopausally
(E) It is also referred to as salpingitis isthmica nodosum

445. A 25-year-old woman complains
of diarrhea and weight loss; her heart
rate is 130 per minute. Head, neck,
and chest x-rays, upper gastrointestinal
series, small-bowel follow-through, and
barium enema all are negative. An
ovarian lesion, discovered during laparotomy, is biopsied (a photomicrograph
of a specimen is shown below) and excised. After her tumor was removed,
the woman's symptoms disappeared.
The most likely diagnosis is

(A) carcinoid tumor
(B) dysgerminoma
(C) embryonal teratoma
(D) endometriosis
(E) struma ovarii

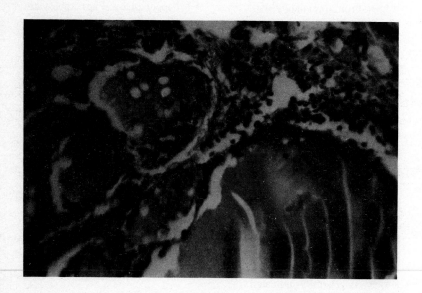

446. Women who have endometrial carcinoma most frequently present with which of the following symptoms?

(A) Bloating
(B) Weight loss
(C) Postmenopausal bleeding
(D) Vaginal discharge
(E) Hemoptysis

447. A 42-year-old woman with cervical carcinoma presents with a central recurrence 2 years after radiation therapy. Regarding pelvic exenteration, which of the following is true?

(A) It is usually possible to preserve the bladder
(B) Surgical mortality is greater than 15 percent
(C) Complications are more common with prior irradiation
(D) The 5-year survival after exenteration is less than 20 percent
(E) The long-term morbidity relates to small bowel obstruction

448. Young women whose mothers took diethylstilbestrol (DES) during pregnancy are most likely to develop which of the following vaginal carcinomas?

(A) Papillary adenocarcinoma
(B) Squamous carcinoma
(C) Carcinoma of the infantile vagina
(D) Adenosquamous carcinoma
(E) Clear cell adenocarcinoma

449. The class of chemotherapeutic agents that is most effective in the management of women who have recurrent endometrial carcinoma is

(A) antimetabolites
(B) hormones
(C) alkylating agents
(D) *Vinca* alkaloids
(E) antibiotics

450. Melanoma of the vulva

(A) constitutes 2 to 9 percent of most series of vulvar cancer
(B) occurs mostly in the fifth decade
(C) occurs mostly in premenopausal women
(D) has an overall survival rate of 70 percent
(E) is nonaggressive

451. Women who have ovarian carcinoma most commonly present with which of the following symptoms?

(A) Vaginal bleeding and anorexia
(B) Weight loss and dyspareunia
(C) Nausea and vaginal discharge
(D) Constipation and frequent urination
(E) Abdominal distension and pain

452. The major mode of spread of ovarian neoplasms is by way of

(A) ovarian veins
(B) ovarian vein lymphatics
(C) pelvic lymphatics
(D) local extension
(E) peritoneal seeding

453. A 54-year-old woman undergoes a laparotomy because of a pelvic mass, which proves to be a unilateral ovarian neoplasm accompanied by a large omental metastasis. The most appropriate intraoperative course of action would be

(A) omental biopsy
(B) ovarian biopsy
(C) excision of the omental metastasis and unilateral oophorectomy
(D) omentectomy and bilateral salpingo-oophorectomy
(E) omentectomy, total abdominal hysterectomy, and bilateral salpingo-oophorectomy

454. Borderline malignant epithelial neoplasms of the ovary

(A) have a 10-year survival rate of 50 percent
(B) show epithelial stratification of two to three layers and cellular atypicality
(C) should be treated with hysterectomy, bilateral salpingo-oophorectomy, and chemotherapy
(D) account for 2 to 3 percent of all epithelial ovarian tumors
(E) should be treated with pelvic and abdominal irradiation

455. A woman is found to have a unilateral, invasive vulvar carcinoma that is 2 cm in diameter but that is not associated with evidence of lymph node spread. Initial management of this woman most likely would consist of

(A) chemotherapy
(B) radiation therapy
(C) simple vulvectomy
(D) radical vulvectomy
(E) radical vulvectomy and bilateral inguinal lymphadenectomy

456. Microinvasive carcinoma of the cervix is diagnosed on a cone biopsy from your patient. All the following statements are true EXCEPT

(A) depth of invasion below the basement membrane should be 3 mm or less
(B) appropriate therapy includes radical hysterectomy
(C) the overall incidence of lymph node metastases is 1.2 percent
(D) lymphovascular invasion should be absent
(E) the presence of confluent tongues of invasion signifies high risk for lymphatic involvement

457. A 55-year-old woman has a 3-cm raised, irregular white lesion at the mucocutaneous junction of the vulva. A sample of the biopsied lesion is shown below. The most likely diagnosis is

(A) tuberculosis
(B) Bowen's disease
(C) Paget's disease
(D) invasive squamous cell carcinoma
(E) fibrosarcoma

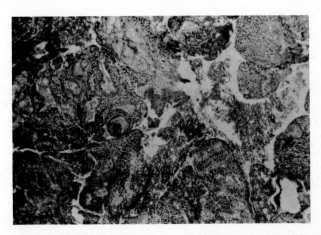

458. The neoplasm most sensitive to appropriate chemotherapy is

(A) gestational trophoblastic disease
(B) ovarian dysgerminoma
(C) Burkitt's lymphoma
(D) endometrial carcinoma
(E) ovarian serous carcinoma

459. Which of the following statements regarding germ cell tumors of the ovary is true?

(A) They peak in incidence after the menopause
(B) They are very different from germ cell tumors in males
(C) They usually are slow growing
(D) They account for approximately 20 percent of ovarian tumors
(E) They rarely cause pain

460. All the following statements about Brenner tumors of the ovary are true EXCEPT that

(A) they generally are benign
(B) they are characterized microscopically by areas of epithelial cells surrounded by mesenchymal tissue
(C) their cells have a characteristic "coffee-bean" nucleus
(D) they tend to grow rather slowly
(E) they rarely are larger than 2 cm in diameter

461. True statements regarding classic or complete hydatidiform moles include that they

(A) occur in approximately 1 out of 120 pregnancies in the United States
(B) are almost always accompanied by theca lutein cysts
(C) have a triploid karyotype
(D) contraindicate future pregnancy because of the high recurrence rate
(E) require chemotherapy for rising or plateauing postevacuation HCG titers

462. A 48-year-old woman presents with a nontender fluctuant mass in her right vulva that causes some discomfort when walking and during coitus and that is consistent with a diagnosis of Bartholin's cyst. What is the most appropriate treatment?

(A) Marsupialization
(B) Antibiotics
(C) Surgical excision
(D) Incision and drainage
(E) No treatment necessary

463. Which of the following statements best describes invasive cervical carcinoma?

(A) Early symptoms include watery, blood-tinged vaginal discharge and postcoital spotting
(B) Periaortic lymph node involvement is present in up to 20 percent of stage I tumors
(C) For early stage disease (I and IIA) survival is better with radical surgery compared with radiation therapy
(D) Recurrent carcinoma is very sensitive to chemotherapy
(E) Intraarterial chemotherapy has had a major impact on survival

464. For patients with operable endometrial carcinoma,

(A) peritoneal cytology is of no clinical value
(B) peritoneal washings reveal malignant cells in approximately 15 percent of stage I tumors
(C) the risk of recurrence is not increased with positive cytology
(D) intraperitoneal P-32 is ineffective when malignant washings are positive
(E) the presence of other good prognostic factors negates the significance of malignant washings

465. Paget's disease is characterized by all the following statements EXCEPT that

(A) it occurs in the nipple and vulva
(B) local recurrences are common
(C) it is often associated with subadjacent adenocarcinoma or squamous cell carcinoma
(D) it often stains darker than the surrounding keratinocytes
(E) surgery is the best treatment

466. Ovarian neoplasms most commonly arise from

(A) coelomic epithelium
(B) nonspecific mesenchyme
(C) specialized gonadal stroma
(D) primitive germ cells
(E) none of the above

467. An intravenous pyelogram (IVP) showing hydronephrosis in the work-up of a cervical cancer otherwise confined to a normal size cervix would mean

(A) stage I
(B) stage II
(C) stage III
(D) stage IV
(E) none of the above

468. All the following statements are true of mature cystic teratomas of the ovary EXCEPT

(A) they are composed of all three germ cell layers
(B) they frequently undergo torsion
(C) they are the most common type of germ cell tumor of the ovary
(D) the most common malignancy found within a mature teratoma is an adenocarcinoma
(E) they usually contain a projection known as Rokitansky's protuberance

DIRECTIONS: Each question below contains four suggested responses of which **one or more** is correct. Select

A	if	**1, 2, and 3**	are correct
B	if	**1 and 3**	are correct
C	if	**2 and 4**	are correct
D	if	**4**	is correct
E	if	**1, 2, 3, and 4**	are correct

469. Clinical symptoms commonly associated with hydatid mole include

(1) nausea and vomiting
(2) hypertension
(3) lower abdominal pain
(4) bleeding

470. True statements regarding cancer of the vagina include that it

(1) is more commonly secondary to cervical cancer than primary
(2) includes a variety of histologic types, such as epidermoid, melanoma, sarcoma, and adenocarcinoma
(3) accounts for less than 5 percent of genital malignancies
(4) is primarily treated with radical surgery

471. Adenocarcinoma of the endometrium can be described by which of the following statements?

(1) It is primarily a disease of postmenopausal women
(2) The average age of affected women is 10 years more than the average age of women who have cervical carcinoma
(3) It has a more favorable prognosis than cervical cancer, with the 5-year survival rate approaching 75 percent
(4) It is increasing in frequency relative to carcinoma of the cervix

472. The spread of adenocarcinoma of the body of the uterus can be described by which of the following statements?

(1) Distant organs, such as the liver, are frequently involved
(2) Dissemination is chiefly by way of the lymphatics
(3) The tumor resembles cervical carcinoma in its frequency of dissemination
(4) Direct extension is an important route of dissemination

473. A patient presents with a Pap smear showing mild dysplasia. The next steps in management would include

(1) hysterectomy
(2) repeat Pap smear
(3) cone biopsy
(4) colposcopy

474. Important prognostic factors concerning ovarian epithelial carcinoma include

(1) extent of the tumor
(2) volume of the tumor
(3) histological differentiation of the tumor
(4) presence of ascites

475. Cervical carcinoma is considered invasive when there is

(1) a breakthrough of the basement membrane
(2) penetration of the stroma
(3) involvement of the lymphatics
(4) involvement of the endocervical glands

476. Which of the following statements can characterize epidermoid carcinoma of the vulva?

(1) It is associated with an increased incidence of epidermoid carcinoma of the endocervix
(2) It is seen less frequently than adenocarcinoma
(3) It tends to develop in women who are older than those affected by adenocarcinoma
(4) It tends to be more advanced when diagnosed than adenocarcinoma

477. Carcinoma of the fallopian tube can be described by which of the following statements?

(1) It is an uncommon lesion, accounting for approximately 0.2 to 0.5 percent of primary genital-tract malignancies
(2) Bilateral involvement occurs in approximately 50 percent of affected patients
(3) Its microscopic appearance can be papillary or papillary-alveolar
(4) It is considered only mildly malignant and is associated with a good 5-year survival rate

478. Nonneoplastic cysts of the ovary include

(1) theca-lutein cysts
(2) pregnancy luteoma
(3) endometriotic cysts
(4) corpus luteum cysts

479. Women are at high risk for endometrial carcinoma if they have which of the following characteristics?

(1) Hypertension
(2) Diabetes
(3) Obesity
(4) Familial history of endometrial carcinoma

480. Evidence in evaluating cell types found in carcinoma of the endometrium suggests that

(1) poorly differentiated adenocarcinomas have a poor prognosis
(2) adenoacanthomas have a poor prognosis
(3) adenosquamous carcinomas have a poor prognosis
(4) adenosquamous tumors occur more often in young women

481. For the management of women who have endometrial carcinoma, intracavitary radium has been employed routinely

(1) as a treatment for women who have ovarian metastases
(2) as a treatment for women who have vaginal apical recurrences
(3) as a treatment for women who have metastases of the pelvic sidewall
(4) as primary therapy for inoperable patients

482. True statements about mucinous carcinoma of the ovary include which of the following?

(1) It usually is diagnosed at a less advanced stage than serous carcinoma

(2) It tends to be unilateral

(3) It tends to be well differentiated

(4) Affected women have a 50-percent chance of surviving 5 years

483. Lichen sclerosis is characterized by

(1) blunting or loss of the rete ridges

(2) development of a homogeneous subepithelial layer in the dermis

(3) a band of chronic inflammatory infiltrate below the dermis

(4) an increase in the number of cellular layers in the epidermis

484. Sarcoma botryoides can be characterized by which of the following statements?

(1) It tends to be multicentric

(2) Its initial manifestation usually is lower abdominal pain

(3) It occurs most frequently in young girls

(4) Cartilaginous and osseous elements are common

485. Meigs syndrome can be described by which of the following statements?

(1) Hydrothorax and ascites are the primary features

(2) It rarely is seen in combination with ovarian fibromas

(3) It can occur with Brenner tumor, thecoma, and granulosa cell tumor

(4) It characteristically is associated with large subserous myomas

486. True statements about ovarian neoplasms in children include which of the following?

(1) They are most often of germ cell origin

(2) They are an infrequent cause of precocious puberty

(3) Coelomic epithelial tumors are usually benign

(4) Tumors of germ cell origin are frequently malignant

487. Epithelial ovarian tumors of low potential malignancy (borderline malignancies) can be described by which of the following statements?

(1) They represent nearly half of all epithelial ovarian tumors

(2) They occasionally are associated with late recurrences and death

(3) They seldom, if ever, metastasize within the peritoneal cavity

(4) They are not associated with destructive infiltration of the ovarian stroma

488. Serous carcinoma of the ovary can be characterized by which of the following statements?

(1) It is the most common epithelial carcinoma of the ovary
(2) It often contains psammoma bodies
(3) It is bilateral in approximately one third of affected women
(4) It frequently is associated with pelvic endometriosis

489. Vaginal carcinoma in women whose mothers received diethylstilbestrol (DES) during pregnancy can be characterized by which of the following statements?

(1) It is most commonly located in the middle and outer portions of the vagina
(2) It classically occurs in women in their teens and early twenties
(3) Electron microscopy has shown that it is müllerian in origin
(4) It occurs in less than 0.1 percent of women exposed in utero to DES

490. Epithelial neoplasms of the ovary can be of which of the following histological types?

(1) Serous
(2) Mucinous
(3) Endometrioid
(4) Mesonephroid

491. Studies show that cervical cancer is associated with

(1) early first coitus
(2) incidence of cigarette smoking
(3) multiparity
(4) use of oral contraceptives

DIRECTIONS: Each group of questions below consists of lettered headings followed by a set of numbered items. For each numbered item select the **one** lettered heading with which it is **most** closely associated. Each lettered heading may be used **once, more than once, or not at all.**

Questions 492–496

For each description that follows, select the ovarian tumor with which it is most likely to be associated.

(A) Granulosa tumor
(B) Sertoli-Leydig cell tumor
(C) Immature teratoma
(D) Gonadoblastoma
(E) Krukenberg's tumor

492. Frequently associated with virilization

493. Frequently associated with endometrial carcinoma

494. Tends to recur more than 5 years following the original diagnosis

495. Calcifications present on pelvic radiographs

496. Correlation between malignant potential and the amount of embryogenic tissue

Questions 497–500

Match each ovarian tumor listed below with the micrograph that correctly exemplifies it.

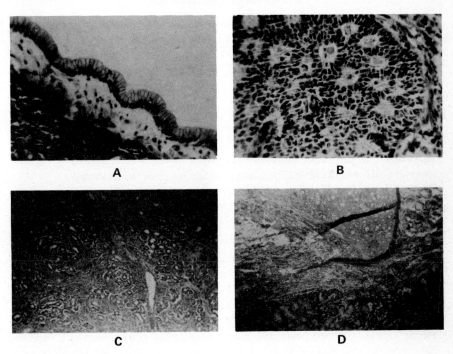

(A) Slide **A**
(B) Slide **B**
(C) Slide **C**
(D) Slide **D**
(E) None of the above

497. Granulosa cell tumor

498. Arrhenoblastoma

499. Benign cystic teratoma

500. Mucinous cystadenoma

Benign and Malignant Neoplasms

Answers

435. The answer is D. *(Morrow, pp 210–214.)* Endometrioid ovarian carcinoma accounts for about 15 percent of all ovarian carcinomas. It is indistinguishable from adenocarcinoma of endometrial origin. Squamous differentiation is common. Approximately 10 percent of endometrioid ovarian cancer is accompanied by ovarian endometriosis, but malignant transformation has not been demonstrated.

436. The answer is B. *(Morrow, p 7.)* According to the International Federation of Gynecology and Obstetrics (FIGO) classification, stage I is carcinoma confined to the corpus, stage II is involvement of the corpus and cervix, stage III is extension beyond the uterus but limited to the true pelvis, and stage IV involves extension outside the true pelvis.

437. The answer is C. *(DiSaia, ed 2. pp 161–167.)* Hysterectomy is the primary mode of treatment for women who have endometrial carcinoma confined to the uterine corpus. External beam and intracavitary radiation have been employed to help reduce central and pelvic recurrences of the cancer. Progestin therapy is used routinely as primary treatment of women who have advanced disease or recurrent carcinoma, and chemotherapy is used for patients whose tumors have failed to respond to other forms of therapy.

438. The answer is D. *(DiSaia, ed 2. pp 149–151.)* Endometrial carcinoma involving the cervix is significant even if present only as microscopic disease. The lymphatic drainage of the uterine corpus is primarily by way of the lymphatics that follow the ovarian vessels. Because involvement of the cervix allows the cancer to metastasize via the parametrial lymphatics, the 5-year survival rate is reduced (regardless of the volume of tumor present) and intense radiotherapeutic treatment is required. Hysterectomy need not be excluded from the management program.

439. The answer is D. *(DiSaia, ed 2. pp 182–184.)* Mixed mesodermal sarcomas are most common. They are discovered most frequently during a histological examination of a leiomyomatous uterus and are often clinically and grossly indistinguishable from benign leiomyoma. A rapid enlargement of a leiomyomatous uterus may be the only indication of the presence of a sarcoma.

440. The answer is B. *(Novak, ed 8. pp 307–310.)* Mixed mesodermal tumors (mesenchymomas) of the uterus are similar to endometrial sarcoma. They are made up of a composite of mesodermal elements such as bone, cartilage, and muscle. The combined incidence of these two types of malignancy is no higher than 0.5 percent of all gynecological malignancies. Although mixed mesodermal tumors occur most frequently in postmenopausal women, one variant, sarcoma botryoides, can develop in young children. Prognosis is poor, with a 5-year survival rate of 26 to 28 percent being the highest reported. Maternal ingestion of estrogen during pregnancy has not, as yet, been associated with the development of mixed mesodermal tumors.

441. The answer is A. *(Kistner, ed 4. pp 196–202.)* Uterine leiomyoma or fibroids occur more commonly in black women and have not been reported prior to menarche. Degeneration—including hyaline, cystic, calcific, red, and sarcomatous—are frequent. Surgery is usually recommended when the uterus fills the true pelvis (12 weeks size). The choice of surgical procedure depends on the patient's age, fertility wishes, severity of symptoms, and suspicion of malignancy.

442. The answer is A. *(DiSaia, ed 2. pp 288–298.)* Ovarian carcinoma, though the third most common malignancy of gynecological origin (after endometrial and cervical carcinoma), is associated with the highest mortality among the common gynecological malignancies. The inability of routine screening tests to diagnose this malignancy in an early stage, in contrast to the efficacy of the Papanicolaou (Pap) smear in detecting cervical cancer, is chiefly responsible for the high mortality. Most patients have advanced disease by the time their symptoms appear. Environmental, cultural, socioeconomic, and dietary factors all may play a role in the development of ovarian cancer.

443. The answer is D. *(Novak, ed 8. p 606.)* Postoperative whole-abdomen irradiation combined with additional radiation to the pelvis has produced the highest 5-year survival rates of any treatment used for patients who have stage II epithelial ovarian tumors. Because ovarian tumor cells tend to exfoliate and spread throughout the abdominal cavity, irradiation of the pelvis alone is insufficient treatment. The liver and kidneys must be shielded during at least part of the external beam therapy, and bowel injury may be a late sequela.

444. The answer is C. *(Kistner, ed 4. pp 191–196.)* Adenomyosis is a common disease of the myometrium occurring in the reproductive years, and more often in multiparas. Most patients present with bleeding and pain. Salpingitis isthmica nodosum, characterized by nodular thickenings of the oviduct, is seen in approximately 20 percent of the patients with adenomyosis.

445. The answer is E. *(Novak, ed 8. pp 490–494.)* The tissue specimen that accompanies the question represents struma ovarii, which is composed of aberrant thyroid tissue that is frequently active and which is associated with mature cystic teratomas. The woman described manifests symptoms of thyrotoxicosis, such as diarrhea, rapid pulse, and weight loss; though not reported, her serum thyroxine levels would be elevated. The pathological picture is characterized by thyroid tissue with large acini filled with colloid.

446. The answer is C. *(Jones, ed 10. p 411.)* Postmenopausal bleeding is the most common presenting symptom of women who have endometrial carcinoma. Because this warning signal is present even in the earliest stage of the disease, early diagnosis and treatment are possible. In fact, approximately 70 percent of affected women have stage I disease when they first seek treatment.

447. The answer is C. *(DiSaia, ed 2. pp 107–115.)* Pelvic exenteration for advanced or recurrent cervical cancer involves removal of the bladder because of its proximity to the cervix. Surgical mortality is less than 5 percent in major centers, and survival varies from 20 to 62 percent. Following irradiation, increased surgical difficulty and poor wound healing contribute to a higher complication rate. Long-term complications are related primarily to urinary diversion.

448. The answer is E. *(DiSaia, ed 2. pp 237–251.)* Young women whose mothers ingested diethylstilbestrol (DES) during pregnancy are more apt to develop clear cell adenocarcinoma than other types of vaginal carcinoma. Although squamous carcinomas are the most common tumors of the vagina, they usually occur in women over 40 years of age. Two rare vaginal carcinomas are papillary adenocarcinoma, which primarily affects older women, and carcinoma of the infantile vagina, which histologically resembles an endodermal sinus tumor of the ovary. Adenosquamous carcinomas usually are found in the uterus and less frequently in the cervix.

449. The answer is B. *(DiSaia, ed 2. pp 172–173.)* Progestins have been employed successfully in the treatment of women who have recurrent endometrial carcinoma. In many series, response rates of 30 to 40 percent have been noted. The most frequently employed agents have been hydroxyprogesterone caproate (Delalutin) and medroxyprogesterone acetate (Provera). Single-agent chemotherapy with nonhormonal agents has produced disappointing responses in patients affected by advanced or recurrent endometrial carcinoma.

450. The answer is A. *(Blaustein, ed 2. pp 48–49.)* Melanoma of the vulva constitutes 2 to 9 percent of vulvar cancer. The mean age of incidence is 54, and most cases occur in the sixth and seventh decades, although 32 percent are premenopausal. It is highly aggressive, and the overall survival rate is only 30 percent.

451. The answer is E. (*Morrow, p 192.*) Approximately 50 percent of women who have ovarian cancer present with abdominal distension, and 50 percent present with abdominal pain. Gastrointestinal symptoms, which occur in about 20 percent of affected women, often are secondary to the development of ascites. Urinary-tract symptoms, caused by the pressure exerted by a rapidly growing mass, and abnormal vaginal bleeding are the initial symptoms of ovarian cancer in 15 percent of affected women.

452. The answer is E. (*DiSaia, ed 2. p 301.*) Peritoneal seeding is the major mode of spread of ovarian neoplasms. Ovarian malignancies also may extend locally to adjoining structures, such as the uterus, fallopian tubes, pelvic peritoneum, bladder peritoneum, and serosa of the sigmoid colon. Although dissemination by lymphatic and hematogenous routes does occur, it is of lesser importance than peritoneal seeding in producing symptoms and eventually causing death.

453. The answer is E. (*Morrow, pp 197–200.*) The survivability of women who have ovarian carcinoma varies inversely with the amount of residual tumor left after the initial surgery. At the time of laparotomy, a maximum effort should be made to determine the sites of tumor spread and excise all resectable tumor. Although the uterus and ovary may appear grossly normal, there is a relatively high incidence of occult metastases to these organs; for this reason, they should be removed during the initial surgery.

454. The answer is B. (*DeSaia, ed 2. pp 272–275.*) Borderline malignant ovarian neoplasms constitute 15 percent of epithelial ovarian cancers. The 10-year survival is 95 percent. Histology reveals epithelial stratification, pleomorphism, atypicality, and mitotic activity. If unilateral, a salpingo-oophorectomy is adequate following a benign biopsy of the contralateral ovary. For bilateral disease or intraperitoneal spread, more radical surgery is indicated.

455. The answer is E. (*Morrow, pp 298–300.*) Women who have invasive vulvar carcinoma usually are treated surgically. If the lesions are unilateral, are not associated with fixed or ulcerated inguinal lymph nodes, and do not involve the urethra, vagina, anus, or rectum, then treatment usually consists of radical vulvectomy and bilateral inguinal lymphadenectomy. If inguinal lymph nodes show evidence of metastatic disease, bilateral pelvic lymphadenectomy is usually performed. Radiation therapy, though not a routine part of the management of women who have early vulvar carcinoma, is employed (as an alternative to pelvic exenteration with radical vulvectomy) in the treatment of women who have local advanced carcinoma.

456. The answer is B. (*DiSaia, ed 2. pp 62–66.*) Microinvasive carcinoma of the cervix includes lesions within 3 mm of the base of the epithelium, with no confluent tongues or lymphovascular invasion. The overall incidence of metastases from 751 reported cases is 1.2 percent. Simple hysterectomy is accepted therapy.

457. The answer is D. *(Novak, ed 8. pp 52–54.)* The woman described in the question has invasive squamous cell carcinoma of the vulva, with penetration below the basement membrane. The squamous epithelial cells have an irregular shape and an abnormal nuclear-cytoplasmic ratio and show an increased number of mitotic figures. Tuberculosis of the vulva is characterized by multinucleated giant cells; tissue with Bowen's disease does not show invasion below the basement membrane; and Paget's disease of the vulva, which is rare, is characterized by Paget's cells, large cells that have abundant granular cytoplasm and basophilic nuclei.

458. The answer is A. *(DiSaia, ed 2. pp 200–211.)* Gestational trophoblastic disease is the neoplasm most sensitive to appropriate chemotherapeutic agents, such as methotrexate and actinomycin D. Treatment of women who have nonmetastatic gestational trophoblastic disease is almost 100-percent successful and allows reproductive function to be preserved. Cure rates for metastatic disease approach 90 percent.

459. The answer is D. *(DiSaia, ed 2. pp 362–386.)* Germ cell tumors of the ovary most commonly occur in young women, grow rapidly, and often produce significant abdominal pain. There is much homology between tumors from males and females. Germ cell tumors account for approximately 20 percent of ovarian tumors.

460. The answer is E. *(Blaustein, ed 2. pp 547–553.)* Brenner tumors of the ovary, which generally are benign, slow-growing, and asymptomatic, account for 1 to 2 percent of all ovarian neoplasms. Size varies widely; although many are microscopic, some may grow to be quite large (one tumor weighing more than 8.5 kg [19 lb] has been reported). Walthard's rests, which are nests of epithelial cells surrounded by mesenchymal tissue, are diagnostic of Brenner tumor. Nuclei of the epithelial cells are grooved longitudinally and, as a result, are referred to as "coffee-bean" nuclei.

461. The answer is E. *(DiSaia, ed 2. pp 192–200.)* In the United States, hydatidiform moles accur in about 1 of 1200 pregnancies. Enlarged theca lutein cysts are present in up to 15 percent. Most have a normal 46,XX karyotype and the recurrence rate is about 17 percent, giving a good chance for normal future pregnancies. Chemotherapy is indicated for rising or plateauing titers or evidence of metastases.

462. The answer is C. *(Blaustein, ed 2. p 26.)* Although rare, adenocarcinoma of Bartholin's gland has to be ruled out in women over 40 years of age who present with Bartholin's cyst. The appropriate treatment in these cases is surgical excision of the Bartholin's gland for a close pathological examination. In cases of abscess formation, both marsupialization of the sac and incision with drainage with appropriate antibiotics are accepted modes of therapy. In the case of the asymptomatic Bartholin's cyst, no treatment is necessary.

463. The answer is A. *(DiSaia, ed 2. pp 68–105.)* Cervical cancer frequently presents with a watery discharge and postcoital spotting. Surgical staging by the Gynecologic Oncology Group has revealed periaortic node involvement in 5.6 percent of stage I lesions. Five-year survival rates of approximately 90 percent are achieved with either surgery or radiation for early stage disease. Intraarterial chemotherapy has not improved the poor response to chemotherapy.

464. The answer is B. *(DiSaia, ed 2. pp 158–159.)* Peritoneal washings are positive in approximately 15 percent of patients with stage I endometrial cancer. Patients with positive cytology have a three- to fourfold higher risk of recurrence. The presence of malignant peritoneal washings negates other good prognostic factors. Intraperitoneal P-32 has been efficacious in decreasing recurrences in patients with positive washings.

465. The answer is D. *(Blaustein, ed 2. pp 42–45.)* Paget's cells often present singly or in nests, and their pale cytoplasm easily differentiates them from surrounding keratinocytes. Paget's cells should be a clue to underlying breast carcinoma or squamous cell carcinoma of the genital region. Paget's disease commonly occurs in the nipple and vulva and local recurrences are common. The recommended treatment is surgery.

466. The answer is A. *(Morrow, pp 201–202.)* Ovarian neoplasms arise more commonly from coelomic epithelium than from any other source. Many tumors of this group include epithelium that histologically resembles endocervical, endometrial, or fallopian-tube epithelium (giving rise, respectively, to mucinous, endometroid, and serous carcinomas). Other, less common ovarian tumors of coelomic epithelial origin include mesonephroid carcinoma, Brenner tumors, mixed mesodermal tumors, and carcinosarcomas. Epithelial tumors frequently contain mixed cell types; categorization of these tumors is according to the cell type that predominates.

467. The answer is C. *(Morrow, p 78.)* By definition a positive IVP would mean extension to the pelvic side wall and thus a stage III carcinoma, specifically stage IIIb. Such staging applies even if there is no palpable tumor beyond the cervix.

468. The answer is D. *(Blaustein, ed 2. pp 632–637.)* Mature cystic teratomas or dermoid cysts are the most common type of germ cell ovarian tumor. All three germ cell layers (endoderm, ectoderm, and mesoderm) are present as well as a small nodule known as Rokitansky's protuberance. Torsion is the most frequent complication. The most common malignancy within a mature cystic teratoma is a squamous cell carcinoma.

469. The answer is E (all). *(Morrow, p 329.)* Hydatid moles are suspected and diagnosed by symptoms that include nausea and vomiting, hypertension from toxemia, lower abdominal pain, and bleeding. Further data include a uterine size large for dates and a characteristic honeycomb pattern on ultrasound. Karyotype of molar tissue reveals 46,XX.

470. The answer is A (1, 2, 3). *(DiSaia, ed 2. pp 237–244.)* Primary cancer of the vagina accounts for approximately 1 to 2 percent of genital malignancies and is treated primarily with radiation therapy. Secondary involvement of the vagina by other tumors is more common than primary vaginal cancer. Tumors of several different histologic types are encountered.

471. The answer is E (all). *(Blaustein, ed 2. pp 330–333.)* Although the carcinogenesis of endometrial cancer is still in dispute, several facts regarding its incidence are clear. The disease primarily affects women who have passed the menopause; on the average, endometrial cancer appears 10 years later than the onset of cervical carcinoma. The fact that the frequency of this condition has been increasing certainly is due in part to the increased life span of American women. Most studies have revealed a 5-year survival rate of about 75 percent for women who have endometrial cancer.

472. The answer is C (2, 4). *(Blaustein, ed 2, pp 330–333.)* Although the most common route of dissemination of adenocarcinoma of the body of the uterus is the lymphatics, this tumor spreads much less often than cervical malignancies and only rarely affects distant organs. Nearby surface structures are affected more frequently, and the cervix, bladder, and rectum can become involved in advanced cases. Direct extension, though not as common as lymphatic dissemination, also is important.

473. The answer is C (2, 4). *(Blaustein, ed 2. pp 172–173.)* The management of the patient in question would require a repeat Pap smear and biopsies to rule out invasive disease before any treatment is undertaken, especially the more invasive procedures. The biopsies should be colposcopically directed.

474. The answer is E (all). *(Morrow, pp 231–232.)* The extent (or stage) and the volume of a tumor are probably the most important prognostic considerations in the management of women who have ovarian epithelial carcinoma. However, on a stage-for-stage basis, women who have well-differentiated tumors have better prognoses than women who have poorly differentiated tumors. The presence of ascites or peritoneal washings that are cytologically positive for malignant cells decreases the 5-year survival of affected women.

475. The answer is A (1, 2, 3). *(Blaustein, ed 2. pp 200–207.)* Carcinoma of the cervix is considered to be invasive when the basement membrane has been pierced, allowing cancer cells into the stroma. Histological evidence of abnormal cell maturation and presence of cancer cells in the lymphatics also indicates invasive disease. Involvement of endocervical glands is not indicative of invasion.

476. The answer is B (1, 3). *(Morrow, pp 287–288.)* Epidermoid carcinoma, the most common variety of vulvar cancer, usually is diagnosed at a less advanced stage than adenocarcinoma, which is a rare tumor that most often arises from Bartholin's glands. Epidermoid carcinoma tends to affect women who, on the average, are older than those affected by adenocarcinoma. Women who have epidermoid carcinoma of the vulva have been noted to have an increased incidence of epidermoid carcinoma of the cervix.

477. The answer is B (1, 3). *(Blaustein, ed 2. pp 409–410.)* Because affected women have a low 5-year survival rate, primary tubal carcinoma is thought to be highly malignant; this relationship, however, may be due more to delayed discovery of the tumor than to its malignant potential. Primary tubal carcinoma accounts for only 0.2 to 0.5 percent of primary malignancies of the genital tract. Microscopically, these tumors present a papillary or papillary-alveolar pattern. Bilateral involvement occurs in about one-fourth of affected women.

478. The answer is E (all). *(Morrow, p 188.)* Corpus luteum cysts represent normal functional cysts. Theca-lutein cysts are follicular cysts with luteinization of the thecal cells. Pregnancy luteoma is a nodular hyperplasia of ovarian lutein cells. Endometriotic cysts are the result of cyclic hemorrhage into a focus of ovarian endometriosis.

479. The answer is E (all). *(DiSaia, ed 2. pp 146–147.)* Endometrial carcinoma tends to occur in obese, diabetic women who undergo late-onset menopause and are nulliparous or have low parity. Other factors that may predispose to endometrial carcinoma include hypertension, cancer at other sites (e.g., ovary and breast), and familial history of this malignancy.

480. The answer is B (1, 3). *(Jones, ed 10. pp 405–410.)* Recent evidence suggests that adenosquamous carcinoma of the endometrium has a poorer prognosis than either adenocarcinoma or adenoacanthoma of the endometrium. It has yet to be resolved whether the poorer prognosis associated with adenosquamous lesions is due to the population of malignant squamous cells or to the poorly differentiated adenomatous elements, which normally carry a poor prognosis. Adenoacanthoma, which is characterized by benign metaplasia of squamous epithelium, has a prognosis similar to that of other adenocarcinomas of the endometrium. Adenosquamous tumors tend to occur more frequently in older women.

481. The answer is C (2, 4). *(DiSaia, ed 2. p 167.)* Intracavitary radium has been successfully employed as the primary mode of therapy for women who have sur- gically inoperable endometrial cancer and have small uteri with a well-differentiated tumor. Vaginal apical recurrences occur in 10 to 15 percent of affected women who were treated by hysterectomy alone; this incidence can be reduced significantly with the use of intravaginal radium. Because the effectiveness of intracavitary radium rapidly decreases as tissue depth increases, it is not a satisfactory treatment for women who have ovarian or pelvic sidewall metastases.

482. The answer is E (all). *(Blaustein, ed 2. pp 529–530.)* Mucinous carcinomas of the ovary usually are diagnosed at an earlier stage than serous carcinomas and tend to be histologically well differentiated. This combination of diagnosis at an early stage (when the tumors frequently are unilateral) and well-differentiated his- tological appearance is probably the reason that women who have mucinous carci- noma have a better 5-year survival rate than women affected by serous carcinoma. Mucinous tumors of the ovary, which are less common than serous lesions, usually are lobulated and may grow to enormous proportions.

483. The answer is A (1, 2, 3). *(Blaustein, ed 2. pp 37–39.)* Lichen sclerosis was formerly termed lichen sclerosis et atrophicus, but recent studies have concluded that atrophy does not exist. Mitotic figures are rare, however. There is an associated decrease in the number of cellular layers as well as a loss in the number of melan- ocytes. Mechanical trauma has produced bullous areas of lymphedema and lacunae filled with erythrocytes, and ulcerations may be seen. It is not a premalignant lesion.

484. The answer is B (1, 3). *(Morrow, pp 282–283. Romney, ed 2. p 379.)* Sarcoma botryoides, a rare and highly malignant tumor, is characterized grossly by a polypoid mass that can expand to occupy the entire vagina and frequently protrudes through the vaginal introitus. The usual presenting symptom is vaginal discharge or bleeding. Sarcoma botryoides, which occurs most frequently in young girls, is usu- ally multicentric in origin. Cartilaginous and osseous elements are not commonly found, although rhabdomyoblastic elements are. Extensive surgery (extenteration), without which death will result, can extend the survival rate to several years.

485. The answer is B (1, 3). *(Blaustein, ed 2. p 588.)* Hydrothorax and ascites are the characteristic features of Meigs syndrome. It is believed that fluid accumu- lates in the thorax by permeating through diaphragmatic lymphatics. First described in association with ovarian fibromas, Meigs syndrome also can be seen in combi- nation with Brenner tumors, thecomas, granulosa cell tumors, and other solid ovarian tumors; large subserous myomas, however, are not associated with development of this syndrome.

486. The answer is E (all). *(Morrow, p 257–259.)* Most ovarian neoplasms in children are of germ cell origin, and about half of these tumors are malignant. Functioning ovarian tumors have been reported to produce precocious puberty in about 2 percent of affected patients. Epithelial tumors of the ovary, which are quite rare in prepubertal girls, are benign in approximately 90 percent of all cases.

487. The answer is C (2, 4). *(Morrow, pp 207–208.)* Epithelial ovarian tumors of low potential malignancy represent 15 percent of all epithelial ovarian tumors. Although they do not infiltrate destructively into the ovarian stroma, these borderline malignancies have been associated with late recurrences and death and may metastasize throughout the peritoneal cavity. Histologically, these tumors demonstrate proliferative activity, abnormal mitoses, and nuclear abnormalities. Ten-year survival rates of women who have stage I tumors of low potential malignancy have been reported to be 95 percent.

488. The answer is A (1, 2, 3). *(Morrow, pp 208–209.)* Serous carcinoma is the most common epithelial tumor of the ovary. Psammoma bodies can be seen in approximately 30 percent of these tumors; and bilateral involvement characterizes about one third of all serous carcinomas. Although mesonephroid carcinomas tend to be associated with pelvic endometriosis, a similar association has not been demonstrated for serous carcinomas.

489. The answer is E (all). *(Blaustein, ed 2. pp 69–71, 105–108.)* A number of young women whose mothers were treated with DES during pregnancy (particularly before the eighteenth week of gestation) have been found to have andenocarcinoma of the vagina. The tumors of these women, who generally are in their late teens or early twenties, usually are located in the middle third or outer third of the vagina. Microscopic examination reveals that the malignancies are clear cell tumors with papillary projections; when viewed by electron microscopy, these tumors show evidence of a müllerian origin.

490. The answer is E (all). *(Blaustein, ed 2. pp 511–512.)* Epithelial neoplasms, which constitute 75 to 80 percent of all primary ovarian cancers, may be of the following histological types: serous, mucinous, endometrioid, and mesonephroid. These types may be thought of as forms of differentiated mesotheliomas. Serous lesions are the most common variety of ovarian cystomas. Mucinous tumors may become large enough to fill the abdomen. The prognosis is good for women who have endometrioid lesions, which metastasize only infrequently, and are not considered to be very malignant. Pure mesonephroid tumors are rare.

491. The answer is B (1, 3). *(Novak, ed 8. pp 297–301.)* The main risk factors of cervical cancer include early exposure to coitus, especially with multiple partners, multiparity, and infection with herpes simplex virus type 2 and other viruses. The role of oral contraceptives has not been established.

492–496. The answers are: 492-B, 493-A, 494-A, 495-D, 496-C. *(Morrow, pp 244, 249–252.)* Sertoli-Leydig cell tumors, which represent less than 1 percent of ovarian tumors, may produce symptoms of virilization. Histologically, they resemble fetal testes; clinically, they must be distinguished from other functioning ovarian neoplasms as well as from tumors of the adrenal glands. Recurrences of Sertoli-Leydig cell tumors, which seem to have a low malignant potential, usually appear within 3 years of the original diagnosis.

Granulosa and theca cell tumors often are associated with excessive estrogen production, which may cause pseudoprecocious puberty, postmenopausal bleeding, or menorrhagia. These tumors are associated with endometrial carcinoma in 15 percent of patients. Because these tumors are quite friable, affected women frequently present with symptoms caused by tumor rupture and intraperitoneal bleeding. Granulosa tumors are low-grade malignancies that tend to recur more than 5 years after the initial diagnosis. Because their malignant potential is impossible to predict histologically, long-term follow-up is mandatory for these patients. Recurrences have been reported as late as 33 years after the original diagnosis.

Gonadoblastomas frequently contain calcifications that can be detected by plain radiography of the pelvis. Women who have gonadoblastomas often have ambiguous genitalia. The tumors are usually small and, in one third of affected women, bilateral.

The malignant potential of immature teratomas correlates with the degree of immature or embryonic tissue present. The presence of choriocarcinoma can be determined histologically as well as by human chorionic gonadotropin (HCG) assays. The presence of choriocarcinoma in an immature teratoma worsens the prognosis.

Krukenberg's tumors are typically bilateral, solid masses of the ovary that nearly always represent metastases from another organ, usually the stomach. They contain large numbers of signet-ring adenocarcinoma cells within a cellular hyperplastic but nonneoplastic ovarian stroma.

497–500. The answers are: 497-B, 498-C, 499-D, 500-A. *(Blaustein, ed 2. pp 525–528, 582–587, 627–645, 693.)* Granulosa cell tumors show considerable microscopic variation. In most instances constituent cells resemble granulosa cells; and Call-Exner bodies, which are small liquefied cysts common in granulosa cells, may be observed in the better-differentiated forms of the tumor.

Arrhenoblastomas are malignant, masculinizing ovarian tumors. Testicular structures may be present (in the accompanying micrograph, testicular-like tubules can be observed). Reinke crystalloids also are often noted.

Benign cystic teratomas are the most common type of ovarian teratomas. The presence of sebaceous glandular elements is common; bone, cartilage, hair follicles, and skin also are frequently encountered.

Mucinous cystadenomas are characterized by the presence of the familiar, columnar, mucin-producing cell lining of the cyst cavity. No evidence of malignancy typically is found.

Bibliography

Aladjem S, Brown AK (eds): *Clinical Perinatology*, 2nd ed. St. Louis, CV Mosby, 1980.

American College of Obstetricians and Gynecologists: Suspect rape. *Am Coll Obstet Gynecol Tech Bull* 14, 1972.

Benirschke K: Twin placenta in perinatal mortality. *NY State J Med* 61:4499–4508, 1961.

Blaustein A (ed): *Pathology of the Female Genital Tract*, 2nd ed. New York, Springer-Verlag, 1982.

Burrow GN, Ferris TF (eds): *Medical Complications During Pregnancy*, 2nd ed. Philadelphia, WB Saunders, 1982.

Center for Disease Control: Treatment guidelines. *Medical Letter* 28:23–28, 1986.

Danforth DR: *Obstetrics & Gynecology*, 4th ed. Hagerstown, Harper & Row, 1983.

DiSaia PJ, Creasman WT: *Clinical Gynecologic Oncology*, 2nd ed. St. Louis, CV Mosby, 1984.

Evans MI, Schulman JD: *Prenatal diagnosis: Invasive technique and MSAFP screening*, in Avery GB (ed): *Neonatology*, 3rd ed. Philadelphia, JB Lippincott, 1987.

Gastel B, Haddow JE, Fletcher JC (eds): *Maternal Serum Alpha Fetoprotein: Issues in the Prenatal Screening and Diagnosis of Neural Tube Defects*. Washington, DC, US Government Printing Office, 1981.

Huffman, JW, et al: *The Gynecology of Childhood and Adolescence*, 2nd ed. Philadelphia, WB Saunders, 1981.

Jeanty P, Romero R: *Obstetrical Ultrasound*. New York, McGraw-Hill, 1984.

Jones HW, Jones GS: *Novak's Textbook of Gynecology*, 10th ed. Baltimore, Williams & Wilkins, 1981.

Kase N, Weingold AB: *Principles of Clinical Gynecology*. New York, Wiley, 1983.

Kistner RW: *Gynecology: Principles and Practice*, 4th ed. Chicago, Year Book Medical Publishers, 1985.

Lin CC, Evans MI: *Intrauterine Growth Retardation: Pathophysiology and Clinical Management*. New York, McGraw-Hill, 1984.

Masters WH, Johnson VE: *Human Sexual Inadequacy*. Boston, Little, Brown, 1970.

Masters WH, Johnson VE: *Human Sexual Response*. Boston, Little, Brown, 1966.

Mattingly RF: *Te Linde's Operative Gynecology*, 6th ed. New York, JB Lippincott, 1985.

Monif GR (ed): *Infectious Diseases in Obstetrics and Gynecology*, 2nd ed. Hagerstown, Harper & Row, 1982.

Morrow CP, Townsend DE: *Synopsis of Gynecologic Oncology*, 2nd ed. New York, Wiley, 1981.

Novak ER, Woodruff JD: *Novak's Gynecologic and Obstetric Pathology: With Clinical and Endocrine Relations*, 8th ed. Philadelphia, WB Saunders, 1979.

Ostergard DR: *Gynecologic Urology and Urodynamics: Theory and Practice*, 2nd ed. Baltimore, Williams & Wilkins, 1985.

Pritchard JA, MacDonald PC: *Williams Obstetrics*, 17th ed. New York, Appleton-Century-Crofts, 1985.

Queenan JT: *Modern Management of the RH Problem*, 2nd ed. Hagerstown, Harper & Row, 1977.

Romney SL, et al (eds): *Gynecology and Obstetrics: The Health Care of Women*, 2nd ed. New York, McGraw-Hill, 1981.

Ryan GM Jr (ed): *Ambulatory Care in Obstetrics and Gynecology*. New York, Grune & Stratton, 1980.

Sciarra JJ (ed): *Gynecology and Obstetrics*, 51st ed. Hagerstown, Harper & Row, 1986.

Smith DW: *Recognizable Patterns of Human Malformation: Genetic, Embryologic, and Clinical Aspects*, 3rd ed. Philadelphia, WB Saunders, 1982.

Speroff L, Glass RH, Kase NG: *Clinical Gynecologic Endocrinology and Infertility*, 3rd ed. Baltimore, Williams & Wilkins, 1983.

Therman E: *Human Chromosomes: Structure, Behavior, Effects*. New York, Springer-Verlag, 1980.

Thompson JS, Thompson MW: *Genetics in Medicine*, 4th ed. Philadelphia, WB Saunders, 1985.

Wilson JD, Foster DW (eds): *Williams' Textbook of Endocrinology*, 7th ed. Philadelphia, WB Saunders, 1985.

Wynn RM: *Obstetrics and Gynecology: The Clinical Core*, 3rd ed. Philadelphia, Lea & Febiger, 1983.